Replenish

Replenish

Diet Mind & Brain Diet

*Using Diet and Meditation to Help Relieve
Common Mood and Neurological Disorders*

Bhuvana Mandalapu, M.D.

iUniverse, Inc.
Bloomington

Replenish
Diet Mind & Brain Diet

iUniverse books may be ordered through booksellers or by contacting:

iUniverse
1663 Liberty Drive
Bloomington, IN 47403
www.iuniverse.com
1-800-Authors (1-800-288-4677)

Because of the dynamic nature of the Internet, any web addresses or links contained in this book may have changed since publication and may no longer be valid. The views expressed in this work are solely those of the author and do not necessarily reflect the views of the publisher, and the publisher hereby disclaims any responsibility for them.

Any people depicted in stock imagery provided by Thinkstock are models, and such images are being used for illustrative purposes only.

Certain stock imagery © Thinkstock.

ISBN: 978-1-4759-8413-2 (sc)
ISBN: 978-1-4759-8414-9 (e)

Printed in the United States of America

iUniverse rev. date: 04/19/2013

The secret formula to happiness is in your heart.
The secret of success is within "the treasure chest of your own troubles".
The path of effort to attain happiness and success as yours is the greatest joy.
The key is moderation.
Ignite it with meditation.

DEDICATION

To my teachers and patients, who gave me the opportunity to learn and serve. My sincere thanks to my friends and family, especially to Dr. Lam, Chandra, Chava, Pamulapati and Mr. & Ms. Murty for guiding me through the difficult times with their brilliant patience.

PREFACE

While not becoming ill is a blessing, a miraculous, easy and complete recovery is a greater blessing. A disease or illness will still make an solid, permanent impression on us, but if no harm is done, it is well and good. What has passed is in the past.

Unfortunately, most mood disorders, and especially neurological disorders, are chronic. They can be debilitating, with permanent, lingering consequences that pull us down day by day like enemies living within us. While modern medical sciences are trying to relieve the symptoms, that burden us, a full recovery is the ideal goal, We have two good friends that will help us on the journey towards a good and quicker recovery. They are with us all the time, helping your body and motivating your reason for betterment. To recover well and quickly, to become more functional, and to be your self as were before, or at least to slow down the more functional decline, these two key friends will give much more than expected.

They are ideal, fair and balanced diet and the daily Meditation. "Replenish"" is about knowing the healthy diet added to the meditation practices to help harmony between the conscious and subconscious minds and ultimately to make us Recoup more, faster to recover previous functional status.

It is about to prove that when we practice consistently with basic concepts of "don't give-up" and "moderation in practice" So that, we will achieve goals far more than what we thought before. Finally, "Replenish" is about rebuilding your mind by development of your brain and mind capabilities, with the benefit of constant but moderate practice with meditation and ideal dietary practices.

The current medical advancements are pioneering, in Deep brain stimulation, magnetic stimulation and ultrasound techniques to neuromodulate the Brain and Mood. Science is in the pursuit of replacing the circuits, restoring the communications and regaining the lost function of the Brain. Meanwhile, the meditation and dietary practices contribute much to that and also add to the pursuit of consistent happiness. We are the noun, verb and essence of our own life. Give a memorable and exceptional ability to it.

A WORD FROM THE AUTHOR

This started as a 'booklet' to spread along a neuro device that is useful in neurological and mood disorders. Curiosity grew too, and the booklet became "Replenish" instead. Hopefully, this information will generate some interest with benefits for a certain section of the readers. This is the collection of my thoughts along with quick guidelines that can assist readers, based on their interest and need.

I want to provide help with this brief message. Please register first as an overview and read again more closely with curiosity. Later, refer to the volume as needed, as a reminder.

There are key concepts of a healthy lifestyle, including eating healthy foods and managing your essential medical needs. Taking care of underlying medical issues such as diabetes, hypertension, high cholesterol, pain issues and other concomitant risk factors, along with your doctor's advice is critical. Taking medications regularly, along with daily physical and mental exercises that occupy your mind with purposeful action is vital. Avoiding the mental activities that waste your energy in a purposeless way is most relevant. Overall, a healthy diet of foods that includes fresh vegetables, fiber, plenty of water, nuts, fresh fruits, adequate amounts of protein, and fat without overdoing it, and limiting red meat are necessary. Limiting your total intake of meat to 2 to 3 times per week, resting well, avoiding unnecessary time in bed and maintaining good, typical sleeping hours are essential.

No diet or mind programs are perfect without maintaining a healthy lifestyle and controlling your medical issues.

By controlling as much as we can, strive also to prepare mind and body to maximize it's potential.

More and more disorders are due to endogenous reasons, including hormonal imbalance in the brain, and familial and genetic disposition. It is true that health sciences are advancing, but at least for now, there is nothing we can do about disorders other than accepting them and treating them. We must treat them with the currently available treatments and other modes of cognitive coping techniques. With good treatment and compliance issues addressed, then maintaining a healthy lifestyle is possible. Staying away from unnecessary stimulants, depressants and destabilizing agents or abusive substances is essential. By following the basic guidelines, we can think about regaining, maximizing potential by additional stabilization and improving the health to the perfect balance. For us, it is a trip to get back to where we were before. Moderation in daily practice and consistency are most valuable to travel with and include meditation in the daily diet to support this journey.

CONTENTS

Part One

Key Slogans & "Pearls of Wisdom" before we start:

Trust yourself entirely.

Ignite your inner strength and positive attitude.

Cultivate your mind for better results

In this ongoing process, all setbacks are stepping stones and blessings in disguise. These add to facilitate the understanding towards opportunities and success.

Imagine yourself with more positive forces.
See as you want to be and beyond.

Be the artist and designer of your life.
Like Darwin's theory of individual variation, each brain is fresh, and only your mind knows how to reach your goal.

"Imagination is more important than knowledge."—Albert Einstein

Whose Job is it? – Anonymous

This is the story of four people, named Everybody, Somebody, Anybody, and Nobody. There is a serious job to be done, and Everybody was asked to do it. Everybody was sure that Somebody would do it. Anybody could have done it, but Nobody did it. Somebody got angry with that because it is Everybody's job. Everybody thought that Anybody could do it. Nobody realized that Everybody would not do it. It ended up that Everybody blamed Somebody, then Nobody did what Anybody could have done.

So please, let that Somebody be the only "body" to do the job and help achieve your goals. Change life and create a better person to yourself and to your beloved family.

Do not become obsessed with the idea of "me and myself" but as far as doing good to your self there is no somebody, anybody or everybody, it is only "you" that can make yourself better.

Health is Wealth

Not having an illness is the best, but when do have one, dealing with it with your willpower is best.

Seek the best possible medical care. Steve Jobs was a genius, yet refused modern medical care for a while. Modern medicine is mainly higher sciences and evidence based. Nothing is wrong with having confidence in modern medicine. Despite great advancements, treatments for all of the diseases are not available yet. Still, the future looks bright with gene therapies, stem cell transplants, and many more different medications continuously in the developmental and trial stages. Health Science has much to offer to future generations.

Do your best to manage and rewire your mind and thoughts to keep your disease in submission and subdued state. A strong mind can manage the disease under better control.

The mind causing the flaring up of symptoms could be as common as the disease itself flaring up with the same symptoms. In many studies, proven that almost 30 % of the symptoms in many cases were psychological, or psychosomatic. If we have insight into the problem and use willpower, we can easily overcome those symptoms and remain symptom free and be more useful and productive.

Keep up with the practice. Determine to fight the disease and keep it off.

Make your company a pleasure to those around.

Discover the power inside. Unlock that potential and become determined to pursue happiness and success. Do not go back in time. Think only forward and see what can change. Do not let your mood and emotions hold back.

Yesterday is gone, and tomorrow is uncertain. Do not know what the future holds, but today, and right now, know that you can do it mindful. Capture the moment, mind and body in one time and space. Practice today to make every step a meaningful and mindful one, It gradually becomes a way to live in "right now, and the ruminations will fade away slowly.
You will start enjoying every movement .

"I know in my heart that man is good, that what is right will always eventually triumph and that there is the purpose and worth to each and every life."
– Ronald Reagan

With daily practice, will see the changes.
Will be more goal oriented and productive.
Will deal with your mood disorders and neurological impairment better.
Your quality of life will recover far better than your original expectations.

Overall, will see the change that always wanted but had not able to get in the past. Your new self will appear to keep forever.
The changes will be reflected in all aspects of your life. Others will clearly notice the changes and will respect.

Object in the air:

The mind that is not trained, not practiced and not maintaining its practice is like an object thrown up in the air. An object will find its way to the ground due to gravity. In the same way, the mind, if not practiced, and not seeking a positive attitude, happiness, and joy in a righteous way, will also lay down. It will fall towards unhappiness and hopeless, lazy ways due to a natural inclination and selection of thoughts towards sadness. To be happy and positive, we need effort and involvement. Without effort and commitment, the mind naturally prefers tragedy, bad thoughts, feelings, and ruminates over them.

"An idle mind is the devil's workshop" H.G.Bohn

Falling fruit:

Even a practicing person that is reaping the rewards of good practice can go back to his old ways due to circumstances make them vulnerable. Just as, a ripened fruit falls down to the ground, a person's habits can lessen. Anyone can fall off as prey due to opposing forces, unhealthy attitudes and thoughts pulling them towards depression, and self-abusive behaviors. During vulnerable times, their self esteem may be injured, can become demoralized due to different states of economic, physical, social scenarios and peer pressures. Some unexpected physical and endogenous behavioral and mental health issues also can do the same, despite taking the medications regularly. Sometimes, circumstances and surroundings make us so vulnerable that we cannot control succumbing to them.

This is the time that a person may need more motivation, and needs to stay in practice to sustain the gains of all these days and years of practice.

Live more consciously during those vulnerable times. When we are emotional, we lose logic. Then all things fall apart and makes us so lonely. Despite having people, counselors, and friends around, you are battling with your own thoughts and emotions. Sometimes, cannot become reasonable and sustain the truth. In those particularly vulnerable times, goal oriented practice to sustain with a positive attitude only can help us further in the right direction.

BRAIN

Neurological Conditions and Their Prevalence

Depression in the United States alone affects more than 17 million Americans each year. That is 1 in 6 people. Anxiety is quite common also. Approximately 450 million people worldwide suffer from some form of mental illness or brain disorder, and one in four people meet the qualifying criteria at some point in their life.

Multiple sclerosis affects more than 350,000 people in US and affects a total of 2.5 million people worldwide.

Parkinson's disease affects 4 to 21 per 100,000 per year.

Essential Tremor: The overall prevalence ratio was 414.6 per 100,000 inhabitants.

Approximately 50 million US adults report having Tinnitus.

Dizziness is common among elderly and associated with functional disability. Dizziness is a common symptom affecting about 30% of the population over the age of 65. Around 12 million Americans over the age of 65 have a dizziness or balance problem that significantly interferes with their lives.

Every year, 780,000 people in the United States have a stroke. Strokes are the most common cause of long-term disability and the third most frequent cause of death in this country. The risk of stroke doubles each decade after the age of 55.

The Center for disease control (CDC) estimates that approximately 1.7 million people suffer Traumatic Brain Injuries annually.

Brain blood and nutrient supply.

There are 2 carotid arteries and 2 main vertebral arteries that become one. The Basilar artery supplies blood to the brain. Although the brain is only about 2% of the total body weight in humans, it receives 15-20% of the body's blood supply. Because brain cells will die if the blood supply which carries oxygen stopped, the brain has top priority for the uninterrupted blood flow. Even if, other organs need blood, the body attempts to satisfy the brain with a constant flow. In humans, the brain uses 15-20% of the body's oxygen supply.

Brain Numbers

The Brain weighs approximately 3 pounds (1250 grams).

The Brain gives rise to 12 cranial nerves which supply the face and head. Four nerves are dedicated to controlling the eyes and vision. Two are for sense of taste, one for smell and one for hearing on each side of the brain.

The brain can survive only 4 to 6 minutes without oxygen before it starts to die.
The time the brain takes before losing consciousness due to blood loss is only 8 to 10 seconds only.

The number of synapses or connections for each neuron in your Brain is 1,000 to 10,000.

There are approximately 100 billion neurons in each normal brain.

The brain is the fattiest organ of the body.

The brain does not have any pain receptors for itself.

The brain areas also have a number system called Brodmann areas. They were defined and numbered by the German Anatomist Korbinian Brodmann. They were based on the organization of neurons he observed in the cerebral cortex using the Nissl stain. For example, the main vision center is called area 17. The main hearing centers are called areas 41 & 42. All of the areas are given a number.

Approximately 90% of the brains cells gets destroyed in the part of the brain called the Substantia nigra before Parkinson's disease symptoms show up clinically.

It is not the brain that is hurting when we get a headache. Brain knows how to avoid and alleviate headaches and other ailments when we train it to do so. It is a complex mechanism that triggers the migraine wave and the blood vessels in head dilate briefly with their pain receptors and create the perception of pain.

It is not true that humans only use 10% of their brain. Each part of the brain has a purpose, and each part helps the other parts, especially the damaged areas. Like a good friend, it is called Plasticity (Extending help). It learns the functions of the damaged brain areas and performs the new duties. (It is like helping a sick family member or taking care of your own kin).

The brain itself is a universe. Anatomically, it sits inside the skull. It weighs around 1250 grams and is actually becoming smaller as we evolve further as modern humans, compared to ancestors. It is unique in structure and function. Just as, the universe is complex with many galaxies, black holes, stars and planets, the brain is complicated.

The brain is comparable to an universe. Just like we started breaking all the complex secrets of the Universe, science is also breaking all the complex secrets of our internal universe - the brain. Many diseases are just like comets, eruptions and planets getting engulfed by the black holes in the universe. Many diseases try to engulf the brain, desiccate, damage, and disrupt it's connections and function. That makes the rest of body and mind non-functional and sub-optimal to achieve goals and ambitions.

Anatomically, the brain is intensely appealing, even in straightforward terms. It has to work every microsecond without any interruption for as long as we are living. Even in sleep, the brain is resting, but still functioning, cleaning it self up. This is done with the blood flushing things in and out, reorganizing the neuronal pathways, and the chemical and neuro hormone secretions getting streamlined for the time we are awake. The brain never stops working.

The brain is fully equipped with plenty of blood supply that delivers oxygen and nutrients continuously. The brain is the only network with plasticity, through it cannot regenerate damaged parts of it.

The main nutrient needed by the brain needs is glucose. Regardless of what we eat, the brain only needs glucose to function.

The brain has several chemicals, hormones and neurotransmitters within itself. It does not need outside chemicals, stimulants like caffeine, alcohol, or other abusive substances. It has the fantastic ability to accept any outside substances and can processes and functions well in limited quantities.

The Brain has few energy stores and relies on cerebral (brain) blood flow to meet it's glucose and oxygen needs continuously. As a result, it is highly susceptible to ischemia (narrowing of the blood vessels). A partially blocked vessel, or an acute blood clot in the blood vessel can cause a reduction or interruption in blood flow in a specific location. A complete lack of blood flow to the brain can lead to death of brain tissue within 4-10 minutes, based on how many other complicated medical conditions one had prior to the brain event. Once blood flow slows cuts down to 20 milliliters/100 grams /minute, neurological symptoms will appear and once blood flow falls to 10 ml or less /100 grams/minute of brain tissue, that part of the brain tissue dies and will never regenerate.

The brain needs nutrients just like other parts of the body, but in different proportions.
The brain holds and makes the mysterious mind of its own and is Unique to every human soul?.

Brain Anatomy

Anatomically, the brain is grossly divided into two halves called the right and left hemispheres.

They control vastly different, specialized functions, along with controlling opposite sides of the body movements and feelings.

Mental abilities are not entirely separated into the left and right cerebral hemispheres of the brain. Some cognitive functions such as speech and language tend to activate one hemisphere of the brain more than the other in certain types of tasks. If one hemisphere gets damaged at an early age, these functions can often be recovered in part or even in full by the other hemisphere by neuroplasticity. Other abilities, such as motor control, memory, and general reasoning are served equally by the two hemispheres.

Right hemisphere

The right hemisphere controls the sensory and motor functions of the left half of the body.

It is mostly responsible for artistic functions, including insight and creativity, artistic skills, music and spatial orientations.

Left hemisphere

The left hemisphere is responsible for controlling the right half of the body, including sensory and motor functions. It is also responsible for spoken language, written language reasoning, scientific functions, and mathematics.

Together, the two hemispheres share a lot of common functions and work in harmony.

The cerebellum likes to know what is happening in any, and all parts of the brain, at all times. It coordinates a lot of activities all at one time. It's main function is balance and coordination. When someone is intoxicated with alcohol, this is part of the brain that gets affected that results in loss of balance, and an impaired state of walking and gait.

The cerebellum is in the back of the head, where as the brainstem is between right and left hemispheres.

The brain stem controls the vital functions of the heart, lungs, sleep and autonomic nervous system.

There are many specialized parts of the brain called the nuclei, which are like strategic locations that control specific functions. They reveal their dysfunction easily when damaged, because of various acquired and genetic causes.

Each nerve cell within these areas, based on their functions, secrete different hormones, called neurotransmitters. They help to signal the cells and generate responses to coordinate the whole brain activity in a harmonious way.

Specific areas of the brain and the neurotransmitters play the main role in the process of disease generation, treatment and outcome.

Additionally, the right and left hemispheres of the brain are separated into lobes - 4 on each side.

The front part is the Frontal lobe, which is responsible for depression, memory, judgment, social interactions, speech and expressions.

The temporal lobes are responsible for memory and speech. This is also the main area where seizures start.

The parietal lobes mainly control motor functioning and processing duties.

The occipital lobes control the vision of opposite eye.

The brain stem controls the vital autonomic functions of the heart and respiration.

The thalamus and hypothalamus control pain, sleep, body temperature, appetite control and other functions.

The main neurotransmitters that brain secrete and depends on their availability for ideal functioning include as below:

Dopamine: Lack of it causes Parkinson's disease.

Acetylcholine: A deficiency causes Alzheimer's, dementia and other diseases, such as myasthenia Gravis.

Serotonin: A deficiency causes depression.

Nor epinephrine: A deficiency causes depression, and anxiety responses.

GABA: A deficiency leads to anxiety and nervousness.

Epinephrine and Nor epinephrine and corticosteroids are responsible for stress reactions.

Relaxation techniques are highly effective for stress reduction. Prescription medications are ok. They can help to cut down the neurotransmitter levels that will help stress.

Memory is not stored in any one particular area of the brain. The hippocampus, temporal and frontal lobes are generally considered memory areas. Memory is an overall function of the brain rather than limited to certain brain cells. That is why, despite brain injury initially cause memory dysfunction, patients eventually recover further due to other brain areas got the memory capabilities.

Remember: The mind and disease have a bi-directional relationship. Disease affects the mind, and the mind affects the disease.

Extraordinary people who suffered from psychiatric illnesses: (wikipedia)

Winston Churchill: November 30, 1874 – January 24, 1965, was a British politician, best known for his leadership of the United Kingdom during the Second World War. He told in his own writings of suffering from "black dog," his term for severe and serious depression

Abraham Lincoln: February 12, 1809 – April 15, 1865, was the 16th President of the United States, serving from March 1861 until his assassination in April 1865.

Vincent van Gogh: March 30, 1853 – July 29, 1890 was a Dutch post -impressionist painter.

Ludwig Von Beethoven: December 17, 1770 – March 26, 1827, was a German composer and pianist.

Michelangelo: March 6, 1475 – February 18, 1564, was an Italian Renaissance sculptor, painter, architect, poet, and engineer who exerted an unparalleled influence on the development of western art.

Charles Dickens: February 7, 1812 – June 9, 1870, was an English writer and social critic.

Charles Darwin: February 12, 1809 – April 19, 1882, was an English naturalist.

Leo Tolstoy: September 9, 1828 – November 20, 1910, was a Russian writer who primarily wrote novels and short stories.

Sir Isaac Newton: December 25, 1642 – March 20, 1726, was an English Physicist, mathematician, astronomer, natural philosopher, alchemist and theologian who had been considered by many to be the greatest and most influential scientist who ever lived.

Sleep /Insomnia Behavior

As humans, we spend one third of life asleep. While every hour of life is precious, sleep duration itself is invaluable. While every person's sleep needs are different, there are many misconceptions among people regarding their sleep, sleep needs, and the quality of sleep.

After childhood, most of us sleep more lightly. Some dream in their sleep throughout life. Deep sleep decreases year after year in both the quality and quantity of sleep. Older people will have some other changes like earlier sleep time and earlier wake-up times. They spend most of their sleep in lighter stages and are more easily awakened..

Inadequate sleep is the most common sleep problem in US despite more than 80 other sleep disorders identified. Only your doctor can evaluate, diagnose, and provide the best possible advice.

Sleep is influenced by many factors, including health problems, physical and mood disorders, environmental, medication effect, and economic and personal issues.

People with the sleep disorders, including difficulties with daytime sleepiness, will find their abilities impaired, as well as their performance and efficiency. They are unable to reach their optimal goals.

They also get different mood disorders such as, irritability, unnecessary conflicts and arguments, as a consequence of a poor night's sleep. In addition to psychiatric problems caused by sleep disturbances; the sleep difficulties can cause flare- up of both physical and psychiatric ailments. Sleep problems can be either with the initiation or continuation of sleep. Sleep deprivation is a significant public health problem now because of chronic and associated risks and consequences.

Insomnia is not easy to treat just with medications.

A person with sleep deprivation can feel a lot of fatigue, and malaise. They may have attention and concentration issues and memory difficulties. They may also suffer from social dysfunction, poor school performance, irritability, daytime sleepiness, lack of motivation and be prone to accidents at the workplace and while driving. They may feel tension headaches, migraines; and stomach upset or irritable bowel syndrome due to lack of sleep. This further escalates into concerns or worries about sleep and makes it difficult to initiate and maintain sleep. This will lead to chronic and non-restoring sleep, furthering deterioration of their physical and mental health.

The consequences of sleep difficulties or insomnia that become chronic are numerous as mentioned above and can lead to various issues. These may include self-medication, alcohol use, over-the-counter and prescription medication use leading to dependence, substance abuse, relapse or worsening of depression. Workplace accidents, absenteeism and daytime difficulties with performance, cognition and even suicide are risks.

As mentioned, medications alone are not the answer. Various cognitive and behavioral therapies can help.

Optimizing food intake, maintaining healthy dietary habits, and timing dietary intake can help optimize good sleep. Additionally, limiting stimulants, or at least stopping any stimulant use by afternoon is helpful. Exposure to the sun in the morning, practicing more sleep hygiene, using biofeedback relaxation stimulus control techniques, meditation, avoiding anticipatory anxiety (like while in bed thinking about your sleep problem) and ignoring the feeling of insomnia are also useful.

Clearing all the misconceptions regarding sleep is particularly useful in tackling insomnia.

Some people perform well with only brief sleep and you could be one of them. They are called short sleepers. There are some famous people who slept remarkably short in their lifetime, yet still performed well.

The following facts can clear some false impressions, and expectations regarding your sleep needs and can solve the sleep worries more quickly.

Normal Sleeper

Most adults have regular sleep needs; functioning better with 7 to 9 hours of sleep. About two-thirds of Americans regularly get this amount of sleep. Children fare better with 8 to 12 hours while elderly people may need only 6 to 7 hours of sleep per night.

One-third of Americans are sleep-deprived, regularly getting less than 7 hours a night, which puts them at higher risk of diabetes, obesity, high blood pressure and other health problems.

Short Sleeper

Short sleepers, about 1% to 3% of the public function well on less than 6 hours of sleep per night without feeling tired during the day. They tend to be unusually energetic and outgoing.

Some popular short sleepers include:(wikipedia)

Napoleon Bonaparte: (August 15, 1769 – May 5, 1821) was a French military and political leader who rose to prominence during the latter stages of the French Revolution and its associated wars in Europe. As Napoleon I, he was Emperor of the French from 1804 to 1815.

Napoleon learned to live with the fact that he was existing on three or four hours of sleep per night. It was said that he used to take catnaps while riding his horse.

Leonardo Da Vinci: (April 15, 1452 – May 2, 1519), was an Italian Renaissance Polymath: painter, sculptor, architect, musician, mathematician, engineer, inventor, anatomist, geologist, cartographer, botanist, and writer. He used to take 15-minute naps every four hours.

Margaret Thatcher: (born October 13, 1925) is a British politician. She is the longest-serving (1979–1990) Prime minister of the United Kingdom of the 20th century, and the only woman ever to have held the post. She sleeps only four hours a night. She has suffered a stroke and is having memory problems.

Winston Churchill: He only spent 6 hours in bed every night. However, he used to take a nap every afternoon that lasted for 1.5 to 2 hours in length.

Michelangelo: Slept four hours per day.

Thomas Edison: (February 11, 1847 – October 18, 1931) was an American inventor and businessman. He developed many devices that profoundly influenced life around the world, including the phonograph, the motion picture camera, and a long-lasting, practical electric light bulb. Edison slept only 3-4 hours a night.

Requirements for sleep vary widely. Most adults traditionally need seven or eight hours of sleep a night, but some adults are "short sleepers" and function well on only three or four hours. Many people overestimate the amount of sleep they need, and underestimate the amount actually getting during a restless night. If loss of sleep impairs ability to function well during the day, it might indicate a problem."

Insomnia

Throughout history, there have been a significant number of extraordinary people who suffered from insomnia. They are from all walks of life and immensely talented. In spite of their inability to enjoy the benefits of a full night of deep, peaceful, relaxing sleep, these gifted individuals had the strength of character to cope up with their sleep problems and achieve extraordinary things in their lifetime.

Every human wakes up many times from the 5-7 cycles of sleep during the night and goes back to sleep. As long as one feels rested, forget about the lack of sleep. Nobody in this world sleeps every night soundly for the same amount of time.

Lighter stages of sleep are the most common in adults. We sleep mostly in Stages 1 and 2. If anyone is craving deep sleep and thinking that they are not sleeping, that is incorrect.

Because of the superficial or lighter sleep that we mostly spend, even a small stimulus, such as a voice, or sound can wake the person up and we will be aware of some things happening around us easily. Still, brain is resting in lighter sleep modes. If anybody takes that as lack of sleep and ruminates over it, can become restless the next day in anticipation of a good sleep every night. It becomes a recurring pattern, an issue of over-tension, and chasing sleep by thinking of insomnia.

Some nights we sleep well and some nights we do not. As long as one sleeps well 4-5 nights per week, we can handle. Some days we will sleep better, and some days we will sleep with less or even with no sleep. We can still perform reasonably well. By taking away the chasing, concern over sleep and by eliminating the anticipated anxiety, things will get better on its own and do not become an issue.

Despite all precautions were taken and all reasons excluded, the true insomniacs may need to use sleep aids a few days per week or even need stronger hypnotic medications. They should choose the right ones that do not cause habituation.

A good night sleep makes feel better by more than 50% in the morning. Even with pain, stress related headaches, fatigue or frustration, all can improve with a refreshing 6-8 hours of sleep in adult normal sleepers.

Some sleep problems are related to other psychiatric problems, alcohol or substance abuse.

Conditions like obstructive sleep apnea, central sleep apnea, Restless Leg Syndrome, Periodic Leg Movements, Narcolepsy and other REM and NREM sleep disorders can be diagnosed and treated well.Loud, irregular snoring and daytime sleepiness are hallmarks of obstructive sleep apnea.

The irresistible urge to move the legs and discomfort are features of RLS (restless legs syndrome) and PLMS (periodic leg movements syndrome), which will create chronic, broken and non-refreshing sleep. Some may need sleep testing before diagnosis and appropriate treatment. Others can be helped with medications alone.

Historical figures with sleep disorders:(wikipedia)

Napoleon Bonaparte: Some reports state he took brief cat naps (micro sleep) while riding his horse. Overall, he used to sleep extremely short periods only.

Winston Churchill: Great Britain's Prime Minister, also suffered from the difficulties of sleeping disorders. Churchill was famous for his afternoon naps and snoring too.

SIR ISSAC NEWTON: known to have suffered from the inability to sleep. He had severe depression.

Thomas Edison: Had immense difficulty in falling asleep.

Benjamin Franklin (January 17, 1706 -April 17, 1790) was one of the founding fathers of the United States. He suffered from severe bouts of insomnia.

Abraham Lincoln and Theodore Roosevelt – both were insomniacs.

Sleep Thoughts of Famous people:

"Fatigue or getting tired is the best pillow" - **Benjamin Franklin**.

"A good laugh and a long sleep are the best cures in the Doctor's book" - **Irish proverb.**

"The worst thing in the world is to try to sleep and not to" - Scott **Fitzgerald.**

"It's a common experience that a problem difficult at night is resolved in the morning after the committee of sleep has worked on it" - John **Steinbeck.**

"The best bridge between despair and hope is a good night's sleep" - **E. Joseph Croossman**

"Sleep is the best meditation"- **Dalai Lama**.

All of these thoughts apply to most of the population. They are known as or called good sleepers or normal sleepers.

The poor sleepers and short sleepers do not need to worry about earlier comments. They do as well as others with short periods of sleep. One has to assess their typical sleep pattern and requirements and satisfy that time frame and sleep hours regularly. They will do as well as any other good sleepers in regards to cognitive and health issues.

Insomnia Prognosis

Short-term prognosis

Depending on the causes, it can be helped by short-term hypnotic agents.

Long-term prognosis

Long term prognosis depends on multiple factors, like maintaining sleep hygiene and avoiding medications that makes one dependent on it. Overall, insomnia is not life threatening. Insomnia often caused by underlying medical issues that cannot be fixed quickly with medicines and devices.

Insomnia

Sunlight affects the pineal gland that secretes melatonin. Melatonin helps us sleep and also regulates temperature. (Thermoregulation).

Maintain uniformly distributed everyday activities. Make time to expos to sunlight in the morning on a daily basis.

Melatonin rises between the evening through the early morning around 4 a.m. And declines thereafter. Light exposure in the evening makes less melatonin and suppresses its production.

Practicing sleep hygiene is beneficial to everyone.
Limit exposure to the sun after 3 p.m.
Keep the lights off in the bedroom during sleep time.
If possible, finish the last meal of the day by 8 p.m. Or even earlier - between 4 and 7 PM.

Do not worry about dreams if they are not part of your sleep. In active sleep, also called REM sleep, dreams are irrational and can be complex. Deep sleep dreams are also called non-REM sleep dreams and are simpler and more realistic. If no dreams still nothing to worry. With the sleep hygiene and meditation the cognitive performance, learning, memory lapses all should improve. The response time also will improve. Persons often underestimate the negative impact of sleep deprivation on cognition and performance.

Many individuals sleep less during weekdays than weekends. Average sleep is 1 to 2 hours less, and younger adults sleep less than seven hours per night. Older adults are more resilient to sleep deprivation than young adults. Usually children sleep remarkably well until adolescence. After that, the delayed sleep phase problem starts, due to their activities. With good sleep, vigilance, alertness and vigor will improve. The tiredness, lethargy, fatigue all will improve. Pain tolerance will improve. The seizures threshold will increase. In fact, sleep deprivation is one of the main triggers for breakthrough seizures. Resistance to infection also will improve with good sleep.

Sleep hygiene techniques and Meditation:

If cannot go to sleep after practicing all sleep hygiene techniques, try doing meditation in the morning for half an hour to one hour.

If cannot maintain consistent sleep and are waking up after few hours, but cannot go back to sleep, then do meditation in the morning and evening.

If cannot sleep after 4 a.m., Do not stay in bed until 6.30 or 7 a.m. Get up and go on with your daily morning activities, including meditation in the morning.

The Brain and Plasticity: Self-healing

Plasticity is the ability to change.
The Rewiring of the brain.
The ability to adapt.

Every normal person has the same amount of brain cells at birth as in adulthood. Those cells grow, reaching maximum size at approximately age six.

Neuroplasticity by definition is the adult's brain's ability to reorganize and adapt, making it able to compensate for environmental changes or disease. The term plasticity is defined as any enduring change in cortical properties as per strength of internal connections, neuronal properties and pattern of representations and controls. It is the re-organization of the brain functions as much as possible, to accommodate the new needs or to regain the function of the lost cells or brain matter.

New discoveries and research prove that the brain has a natural ability to re-develop, re-organize and help the damaged areas far greater than previously believed.

The mind and brain, with the help of coping skills and practices that involves both physical and mental efforts, complementary or supplementary can help neuromodulation and neuroplasticity.

New connections are created each and every time we remember something, or have a new thought. Stronger, more intense emotional connections are linked to memories prompted by repeatedly stimulating our thoughts. Sleep is probably the best time for the brain to consolidate memory, and newly learned things.

Thinking positively is extremely powerful. When we think positively, your brain can overcome 50-70% of symptoms.

Eat right and well, and it will have positive effects on the brain.

Moderation/Balance: Moderation is considered a key part of one's personal development. There is nothing that cannot be moderated, including one's actions, desires and even thoughts.

It is believed that by practicing moderation, one achieves a more natural state, faces less resistance in life and recognizes one's true limits. Taken to the extreme, moderation is complex and can be difficult to accept, understand and implement.

Meditation uses:

In current day and age, along with a disharmonious environment and lifestyles of over indulgence, we need to preserve and protect the health from pain and disease. To have a calm and tranquilizing life, releasing us from anxiety, worries and addictions, meditation is particularly useful.

"Chaos is inherent in all compounded things. Strive on with diligence." - Buddha-

Remember - goals are crucial despite the many obstacles we encounter. Do not give up.

"Replenish" is a small, sincere effort to stress the importance of practice, practice, practice. Consistency is the key to the conquest - to bring their potential out to support and achieve goals.

"I have not failed 10,000 times. I have successfully found 10,000 ways that will not work" - Thomas Edison.

The definition of health is:

"The sound mind in a sound body" How can we maintain and achieve this? If factors that are not in our control are overwhelming the body, brain and mind, how can reach their optimal goals? How to stay comfortable, functional and yet happy with a purposeful soul?

To achieve that, we need to know what our body is composed of, and what it needs, does not need or any abuses that it is receiving on a consistent basis.

The overall representation of one's soul is the expression of the combined efforts of the brain and mind and depends on how carefully we take care of ourselves over time. Throughout life, health is dependent on our practice of mind, brain and body. The physical and mental abuse of the body and mind are like destroying the brain or not maintaining it well. The healthy mind in a healthy body is well suited here.

Mind & Brain Diet

Think positive. Train your brain with positive ways. Doing so, brain can overcome 50-70% of symptoms. Eat well and eat right, and it will have positive effects on your brain and body and gives ultimate pleasure. Rest well and adequately, both physically and mentally. Know that a sensitive balance exists between optimal, balanced functioning of mood, mind and the environment.

A wise woman said " **Hunger does not know the taste. Sleep does not know the Luxury**"

This is particularly true. If we eat only when we are hungry, and sleep only when sleepy, everything is well done. With current societal and, time demands, we have to plan eating and sleeping times. We eat with plenty of choices around us without control.

Moderation/Balance: Moderation is considered a vital part of one's personal development. There is nothing that cannot be moderated. Including one's actions, one's desires and even one's thoughts. It is believed that by practicing moderation, one achieves a more natural state, faces less struggle in life, and recognizes their own true limits. Taken to the extreme, moderation is complex and can be difficult to obtain, but also difficult to understand and apply.

There is no strict diet program that is written in stone. No single program is accurate or wrong, including all of those tried by real popular peoples. Rarely, are people able to continue to certain diets or food specifics. The world had given us so much of a variety. All of us desire to experience the range and consider the choices that we have.

With moderation, we can enjoy the things that we like without any hesitation or regret. Moderation is the way in dietary practices just like any other act or practice. Remember, not too tight, not too loose. The same principle applies as to " not too little or not too much'. Adequate, but moderate choices is the solution for any diet program. Knowing what we need to eat is most useful when practicing moderation. You can be picky about the items that your body and brain need as basic food elements of daily requirements.

The tongue, with its two main functions of speech and taste, is extremely difficult for the mind to control. Control of speech and control of food intake are so complex and require thriving practice. Many of us fail most of the time.

Part Two

Brain Diet

Food, Mind and Brain

"The only way to keep your health is to eat what you do not want, drink what you do not like, and do what you would rather not." —Mark twain.

Until we innovate we may at least improve.

"The body was never meant to be treated as a refuse bin, holding all the foods that the palate demands." – Mahatma Gandhi.

We are made up water and different material products in the formation of proteins, carbohydrates, and fats, along with many minerals and vitamins, all from the ground in one form or another. We function as a human body and brain, with the support of synchronous activity of neurotransmitters and hormones that are made from different elements.

In order to properly maintain body and brain, and to keep them functioning properly, we need approximately 2000 calories daily. The calories are from various forms of foods and are part of the daily maintenance requirements. Ideally, foods contain almost everything that we need on a daily basis. We do eat in excess, and we do taste different foods that may not be healthy. Trying them is different from habitually over eating, or choosing the wrong foods consistently.

Certain health conditions, especially those that are brain and mind related require particular attention. Consuming the right, daily intake of food and nutrients is essential, as is avoiding items, substances, or foods that can hurt them too. To keep the body healthy, along with a healthy brain and mood, use food precautions with constant practice. Additionally, the endogenous, genetic, familial, other exogenous causes predispose us for disease. With good dietary habits, and persistence of practice through meditation, we can cure the disease or limit it's harmful effects and retrieve previous abilities to survive in a healthy state with a healthy mind. Through meditation and by using the capabilities of neural plasticity of the brain and nervous system, we can achieve this.

This is about limiting the dietary advice to only some mood disorders, brain disorders and meditation. For other dietary guidelines, many other resources are available.

What the brain needs:

Good, healthy, caring body: The body is the sanctum Sanctorum of your soul and mind. Care for it well. Respect your brain and soul by respecting your body. Do not indulge in any excess things or actions. Excessive laziness, too much rest, too little rest, too much wear and tear, too much sleep or too little sleep, inadequate eating, excess eating, drinking unnecessary, depressant stimulants, using unnecessary substances and medicines all are disrespecting your soul, brain and mind. Keep everything in moderation and show keen attention to daily activities. Live with flexibility.

Brain Nutrition needs: The brain represents only 2% of the body weight. It receives 15% of the cardiac output, 20% of total body oxygen consumption, and 25% of total body glucose utilization. With a global blood flow of 57 ml/100 grams per minute, the brain extracts approximately 50% of oxygen and 10% of glucose from the arterial blood. Hence, the glucose utilization of the brain is 31 μmol/100 grams per minute. Oxygen consumption is 160 μmol/100 grams per minute.

Glucose can be incorporated into lipids, proteins and glycogen, and it is also the precursor of neurotransmitters such as γ-amino butyric acid (GABA), glutamate and acetylcholine.

The brain performs as the main organizer of various functions for the body. Most are of a cognitive nature or concern the regulation of the motor system.

The energy consumption of the brain is exceptionally high. It consumes 20% of the carbohydrates ingested over a 24-hour period. This corresponds to 100 g of glucose per day or half of the daily requirement for a human being. An average built young person's brain consumes approximately 200 grams of glucose per day.

The brain is exclusively dependent on glucose as an energy source. Lactate and betahydroxybutyric acid can also be considered as substrates but only under certain conditions of considerable stress levels or malnutrition. Also, the brain is separated from the rest of the body's circulation by the blood-brain-barrier. The blood glucose has to be brought there via a specific transporter system.

The brain maintains it's own glucose content and needs. The brain is always supplied with a greater energy share than the body in extreme stress situations. In overweight individuals, the brain's energy distribution mechanism is disrupted. With chronic stress, the energy flux between the brain and the body is diverted, a phenomenon that leads to the development of being overweight.

The brain gets a portion of its energy from ketones. When glucose is less available during fasting or strenuous exercise, there is a low carbohydrate state. In the event of low blood glucose, most other tissues have additional energy sources besides ketones, such as fatty acids, but the brain does not. After the diet has been changed, and the blood glucose stays lower for 3 days, the brain gets 25% of its energy from ketone bodies. After about 4 days, this goes up to 70%. During the initial stages, the brain does not burn ketones since they are an important substrate for lipid synthesis in the brain.

Diets of some Great people

Thomas Edison: Lived last few years of his life consuming milk for liquids. He thought would live longer just with milk. This proved to be wrong, and there was no scientific backing either. Edison was said to have been influenced by a popular fad diet. In his last few years; "the only liquid he consumed was a pint of milk every three hours". He is reported to have believed this diet would restore his health. However, this tale is doubtful. In 1930, the year before Edison died, Mina, his wife said in an interview about him, "correct eating is one of his greatest hobbies.". Edison's last breath is reportedly contained in a test tube at the Henry Ford Museum. Ford reportedly convinced Charles Edison, son of Thomas Edison (the 42nd governor of New Jersey) to seal a test tube of air in the inventor's room shortly after his death, as a memento.

Steve Jobs: (February 24, 1955 – October 5, 2011) was an American entrepreneur and inventor, best known as the co-founder, chairman, and CEO of Apple Inc. Through Apple, he was widely recognized as a charismatic pioneer of the personal computer revolution and for his influential career in the computer and consumer electronics fields. Jobs also co-founded and served as chief executive of Pixar Animation studios. He became a member of the board of directors of The Walt Disney Company in 2006, when Disney acquired Pixar.

Steve Jobs followed strict dietary protocols, but still needed surgical approaches, and that failed to keep him alive. He had dietary habits with an occasional tendency to eat only one or two foods like carrots or apples for weeks at a time. There are other health issues that can arise from adhering to such a limited diet.

Dr. Naka Mats of Japan: The inventor of the floppy disc, CD and many others items. He consumes only 700 calories per day. He follows a strict diet protocol with no coffee, tea or alcohol. He eats only once a day. He uses many brain stimulating devices to sharpen his thoughts. He has the highest number of patents and inventions in his name.

Buddha: He followed no dietary restrictions other than moderation of the total food intake. He ate anything and everything given to him. His last meal contained pork. He ate only once a day, around 11a.m. Most likely, the foods were limited in calories in those days. He enjoyed the food and ate as much as he can in one meal per day. This was especially true on the occasions that he was guest to the villages or to the king's palace. He ate well. He practiced 2 hours of meditation each day, along with a simple walk. This was in addition, to his normal walking from town to town and place to place to teach and deliver sermons.

Buddha followed the principle of moderation with flexibility in every aspect of his life. "Do not pull the string too tight it will break, do not keep the string too loose, it will not give the tune". That is the concept he followed in his every action.

Albert Einstein: March 14, 1879 – April 18, 1955 - He was a German-born, theoretical physicist, who developed the general theory of relativity, one of the two pillars of modern physics, alongside quantum mechanics. While **best** known for his mass-energy equivalence formula $E = mc^2$ (which has been dubbed "the world's most famous equation"), he received the 1921 Nobel prize in physics "for his services to theoretical physics, and especially for his discovery of the law of the photoelectric effect. The latter was pivotal in establishing quantum theory.

Einstein was a vegetarian only for the last year or so of his life, though he appears to have supported the idea for many years before practicing it himself. He said: ", So I am living without fats, without meat, without fish, but am feeling quite well this way. It always seems that man was not born to be a carnivore."

"I have always eaten animal flesh with a somewhat guilty conscience."- *Einstein Archive 60-058*

> "It is my view that the vegetarian manner of living by its purely physical effect on the human temperament would most beneficially influence the lot of mankind".
> – *Einstein's Letter to 'Vegetarian Watch-Tower', 27 December 1930.*

Einstein was a heavy smoker but did not use alcohol in his life.

GANDHI DIET:" *It is health that is real wealth, not peaces of gold and silver".*

"I hold flesh-food to be unsuited to our species" - Mahatma Gandhi.

Gandhi believed that food was an integral part of shaping our consciousness and not just meant to satiate our hunger. He experimented throughout his life to find his 'perfect diet', an experiment that lasted over 35 years. Earlier in his life, he consumed meat only on a few occasions. He stopped eating meat and was a complete vegetarian by 1906.

Bill Gates recently said: "The Future of Meat is Vegan." I do not regard flesh food as necessary for us at any stage and under any clime in which it is possible for human beings ordinarily to live".

Bill Gates: (Born October 28, 1955) is an American business magnate and philanthropist. Gates is the former chief executive and current chairman of Microsoft, the world's largest personal-computer software company. He is consistently ranked among the world's wealthiest people. He has also authored and co-authored several books. Gates has pursued a number of philanthropic endeavors, donating large amounts of money to various charitable organizations and scientific research programs through the Bill & Melinda Gates Foundation, established in 2000.

JK Rowling: Joanne "Jo" Rowling (Born July 31, 1965), pen name J. K. Rowling, is a British novelist, best known as the author of the Harry Potter fantasy series. The *Potter* books have gained worldwide attention, won multiple awards, and sold more than

400 million copies. They have become the best-selling book series in the history, and been the basis for a series of films which has become the highest -grossing film series in history.

To my knowledge, no particular dietary pattern influenced her creativity or imagination. It is self-motivation and spontaneity. We should pursue analyzing her brain images for Einstein like convulsions or any other distinctive patterns.

Tips for Controlled eating

The goal is to reduce the desire. (we eat more than what we need in most cases).

Eat slowly and small amounts each time. Try to use a small fork or spoon if possible.

Do not go for the second serving of the same food item.

Try to limit cooking to just few items per day. (Less variety is good if want to eat less).

Eat consciously without doing anything else while eating.

Just like using the bedroom only for sleeping as part of sleep hygiene, make a habit of eating in one single area, such as the dining table.

Spend less time in the kitchen.

Keep fewer snacks available in the house.

Put food away, in its place, and not in sight.

Keep a food plate or food pyramid poster in the dining room or kitchen.

Chewing

Some research details suggest chewing each bite of food for 30 seconds. While we need not count each time, chewing longer helps aid in better digestion by mixing with saliva in the mouth before it reaches the stomach, where it has already been grinded well. It will be absorbed faster and more. Research has found that chewing longer eventually makes people eat less, and they become thinner.

Precautions given:

Make sure that your diet contains fewer calories.
If your diet is loaded with calories and chew longer, and spend more time at the dining table, it is likely consuming more than necessary. The additional absorption means more and more calories. Normally, healthy people do not tire easily by chewing longer and certainly can complete their plates. People with Myasthenia Gravis or other chewing or swallowing issues may get tired or bored of chewing each bite longer and leave the food. That is not good for them either. I suggest choosing food carefully, limiting the total calories, and if choose to chew longer, add more roughage, such as vegetables to the diet, which will restrict calories. People on some medications who gain weight, despite trying to control the calories, should consider daily portions of

cabbage, cauliflower, broccoli or similar items, which makes the stomach full. They keep the feeling of fullness and make to eat less while on hunger provoking medications.

FASTING

We are not talking about religious fasting.

Basically, this is skipping one meal per week, on the day that you choose. Try not to eat either breakfast or lunch and do not eat anything after the missed meal until the next day. Drink plenty of fluids. This type of limited fasting will not do any harm and does not deprive either the brain or mind of any necessary calories, oxygen, nutrients or minerals. This is like giving the GI tract a rest. It is the same as giving the brain and mind a rest during sleep. It also gives the rest to the body, heart and lungs while resting on the couch or are in bed. Remember Buddha lived healthy and happy life, with just one meal a day throughout his life from age 36 to 84. This will also help to cleanse the GI tract and help the mind and brain to be more alert. This type of limited fasting will not cause any ketosis or hallucinations. Only remarkably few will not have enough storage of glucose in the liver to metabolize during the 10-12 hours of fasting and may not tolerate fasting well. They will do ok by taking their medications as usual and keeping up with clear liquids.

Meaningful improvements in blood pressure, blood lipids, and biomarkers of oxidative stress can occur with no harm done. This will also assist in better digestion on a daily basis.

Do this once a week and also try to skip one additional meal when attend parties or whenever have had an extra large meal. This will help to balance the total calories for that day.

It is easier to give too much to the body, rather than taking away from it.

The excess calories will accumulate extremely fast and are extremely difficult to mobilize and get rid of. Each fasting day will help to mobilize ½ pound of extra calories that are sitting in the fatty deposits. Choose a day out of each week as a fasting day after lunch. This will give be an automated reminder at the beginning of the week. Choose the day that is less demanding, so that you tolerate the fasting without anger and the frustration of hunger. Slowly, that will become a routine habit. This will not let go into any anorexia/bulimia type risk unless have obsessive tendencies for dieting and binging. You can take a multivitamin that day, or on a daily basis, but there is no real need with just one meal skipped per week.

Control excess calories and food intake as much as possible.

Many dishes make many diseases.

Bowel Cleansing

Lot of people, based on the nature of the food that they eat their dietary habits and medical conditions can become constipated on a regular basis, or need to strain frequently. Consequences can include hemorrhoids and other bleeding or abdominal discomfort. Meat lovers are more likely prone to this.

Excessive laxative use can cause habitual constipation.

It is necessary to drink plenty of fluids and eat plenty of fibers. Identify the foods that cause constipation and avoid them. Fruits are preferred, rather than juices. Still, if are prone to constipation, add a stool softener to your daily medications.

If the problem continues after all medical reasons have been ruled out, try a limited dose of laxatives at intervals. Do not make it a habit. To avoid intolerance, try different laxatives, limiting use to once or twice per month. Give the bowel rest by fasting if possible, on alternate weeks. Despite all efforts, some GI tracts become stubborn and autonomic dysfunction intervenes, and they will unfortunately need frequent enemas.

Best times to eat

The maximum acid secretion in the stomach is from 10 p.m. to 2 a.m. It slowly rises again to reach it's peak by 11 A.M. Correlating the two, the best timings for food intake can be achieved.

If there is no other medical condition that requires frequent eating or a need to eat each time with medication, follow these basic guidelines.

It is preferable not to eat anything after 8 p.m. and not again until the morning – 9 a.m. – 11 a.m.

With a busy life, especially mornings, one is already on the road by 6 or 7 a.m. Some people think they need to complete their cereal or other breakfast in the early morning. This may not be a good idea. If one can get a small meal with them, and wait to eat at 9 a.m. Or eat as brunch at 11 a.m., may be the right choice. Otherwise, eat a limited breakfast without juice. Adding a fruit is ok as a substitute in the morning.

During lunch, watch for any high fat /high calorie foods or smoothies. You can take it if you wish.

Once at home after work, it is common to snacks while sitting and relaxing. If can avoid snacking, that is best. Otherwise, use moderation and complete your dinner by 6 – 7 p.m. Try not to eat anything after 8 p.m.

As we discussed, one should be flexible with food, sometimes eating more -, sometimes less. Based on what we have eaten, we can skip some meals without any problem and can compensate that high calorie intake.

Type of foods that the human body and brain needs

Eat Right and reap the benefits.

While proteins, carbohydrates and fats with water are the main building blocks of the body, they are needed on a daily basis in adequate proportions.

Most of the vitamins, minerals we do get on a daily basis are in a balanced diet containing adequate portions of fruits, vegetables, proteins, carbohydrates and fats.

Based on one's health needs, a multivitamin with minerals may be needed on a daily basis. There is no need to consume mega vitamins. If they are lacking in a certain vitamin that can be replaced with adequate doses. There are not tests available to check each and every mineral or vitamin in the body for the levels or deficiencies. Based on a person's symptoms, doctors can check so. Common vitamins and minerals that the body may need to replace when it is deficient are listed below with some clinical importance of their deficiencies noted.

B12 and Folic acid

Dietary intake is the only source for vitamin B12 (Cyanocobalamin) and a folic acid (folate) because we cannot synthesize these in the body.

People who eat an fair and balanced diet that contains both vegetarian and non-vegetarian products can get enough of both, unless have difficulties with the absorption from the stomach with the loss of the unique absorbing cells called parietal cells. Intrinsic factors that allow them into the cells and makes them absorbed from the GI tract and to the body cells and organs. As we age, the GI tract loses the capability to absorb these vitamins, especially B12 (Cyanocobalamin).

Pure vegetarians, who drink only cow milk milk, can have low levels of B12. Cow milk does not have any B12. Dietary supplementation of B12 is essential. Vitamin B12 can be supplemented in therapeutic or maintenance doses if needed.

B12 deficiency can cause many symptoms, including depression, fatigue, memory loss, neuropathy, ataxia, lack of coordination, gait difficulty, disorientation or spinal cord disease. Symptoms can appear two years later after a complete deficiency.

Seeing the blood levels showing a deficiency means B12 has already depleted from the body and is ready to manifest into a clinical symptom or disease.

Usually after age 50 many people lose the ability to absorb vitamin B12 from the food. This is due to the loss of parietal cells and the intrinsic factors in the stomach and colon.

Recognizing this, and treating it may help to some extent, but we will not be able to reverse it altogether if symptoms have already begun. Based on the deficiency, it will be replaced and maintained to prevent further ongoing damage to the brain, mind, body, and nervous system, which can contribute to dementia.

Folic acid - Based on the need, including pregnant females, patients on different medications for other diseases will require additional supplementation. Full deficiency can lead to fatigue and depression. Folic acid is essential for normal brain functioning.

Blindly consuming mega vitamins on a daily basis may not be a good idea. Especially with Vitamin A, Vitamin D, Vitamin E and Vitamin K, which can cause a problem called hypervitaminosis. It has its' own consequences with different symptoms and diseases.

Vitamin B6 plays a role in the synthesis of serotonin, which has linked to depression. The various medications used as antidepressants are called selective serotonin receptor inhibitors (SSRI'S). The deficiency can also affect the ability to release oxygen from the RBC to the cells for proper functioning. Based on the needs, this can be replaced. In older adults, the requirement may be higher.

Vitamin C is also essential as an antioxidant and for adequate brain functioning. It is especially beneficial to take adequate amounts including the elderly. Vitamin C is prevalent in all citrus fruits, and we get more than adequate amounts with a daily balanced diet.

Vitamin B2 is important in the process of energy production to the body. It's also needed for the proper functioning of vitamin B6.

Often elderly people lack it, and daily multivitamin supplementation is probably necessary. Studies showed elderly people living alone consumed up to 25% less than the recommended daily intake of vitamin B2 containing foods. Around 10% of them did show deficiency, that can be helped by replacing as needed.

Vitamin D With people spending less and less time in the sun and the elderly staying indoors - mostly in nursing homes and assisted living facilities, they are not getting enough sun. They are becoming more and more deficient in vitamin D. It causes not only osteoporosis and weak bones, but cognitive issues as well, along with a higher risk for heart disease and types of cancers. There are good evaluation and replacement therapies available.

Vitamin K: Usually, we do not need this as a separate supplement. All of the green, leafy vegetables have this in adequate amounts. People who are on a blood thinner called Coumadin (Warfarin), need to take some precautions regarding excess intake of vitamin K. Your doctor has the best advice regarding the types of vegetables and the quantities to consume if taking Coumadin.

Minerals

We do get adequate amounts of micronutrients and minerals in daily balanced food plate. The micronutrients include the selenium Zinc, Chromium, Nickel, copper, calcium, Iron and a few other.

The other appropriate minerals we all consume daily include magnesium, calcium, sodium in the form of salt, and potassium.

As doctors, we can help to guide with the body requirements for sodium, potassium based on health conditions and medications that are on.

The minerals like **magnesium** can get low because of decreased absorption from the GI track. Magnesium is the one of the necessary minerals in the process of energy production by the body. Based on need, doctor should replace it rather than taking daily the magnesium containing supplements which can harm patients with kidney disease. It can cause problems if there is too much magnesium in the body and if kidneys cannot handle to remove.

Another mineral or metal is **Iron**. We get so often low which causes iron deficiency anemia. While there are many other types of anemia, iron deficiency is the most common. There are blood tests available to find out all the other causes and confirm iron deficiency to treat.

Pregnant women or losing a lot of blood with menstrual cycles, they quite commonly get deficient in iron and need replacement therapy. This can cause swelling of the legs, craving for non-food items including ice and clay.

Copper : Is a mineral that is linked to both psychiatric and brain disorders, especially Wilson's disease, which causes neuropsychiatric problems. It plays a major role in the functioning of serotonin. It is also important in maintaining proper brain functioning, energy production process. It also helps in the synthesis of nerve cell sheaths called myelin. This is not linked as the cause of multiple sclerosis, which happens because of destruction of myelin called demyelination. There are adequate testing methods to treat properly, rather than taking inappropriately in the form of mega vitamins with the minerals.

Remember, balanced diet should have mostly what we need. Based only on the need we have to replace rather than blindly taking mega vitamins or other minerals. Vitamins in excess quantities will get us into trouble with the hypervitaminosis. Other issue is that body liver or kidney's can not handle too much of minerals. Again, moderation is the key term here to practice.

Few words on Spices and other of Neurological interest

Dark chocolate has Flavonoids that help to improve memory.

Spices Turmeric, garlic, and ginger found useful for many reasons and have been in use for millenniums. No harm noted and no calories.

Sprinkle turmeric on any food just like in amounts of salt like 2grams(maximum 10-12 grams or more). This contains a chemical by name curcumin that helps memory and pain relief. While more research is ongoing for its uses in Alzheimer's, no adverse effects were noted with daily usage as a food additive. No taste change, only color may change to slight yellowish. Found to have uses in fighting the immune system helps to retain memory. Widely available as powder and can buy in any food store.

Garlic everybody knows about its benefits and available as many forms. Fresh garlic can be used in dishes on a daily basis. Slightly smells through the sweat excretion. Some people cannot take the smell. Found to have benefits for both neurological and cardiac health.

Ginger available as a fresh or dry powder. Can be used in any dish just like black pepper. The fresh ginger is spicy. For health reasons it can be used as dry powder and just sprinkle on food like salt and pepper. Thought to be good for memory, it may cut down chronic pain, migraines and fibromyalgia related pain as well.

Green Tea Recent research indicates hints of Green tea to protect against Alzheimer's disease(AD) with its antioxidant effects and by reducing plaque formation in the brain.

Food Plate(choose my plate.gov)
We are getting everything that we need

If we follow the food plate/food pyramid recommendations, we are getting everything that we need with the supplement as needed or most people can take a multivitamin on a daily basis. One can consume alcohol in moderation. This is an optional recommendation, not for everyone. Also, there is no reason for the human body to drink alcohol. But if someone likes and enjoys it in different varieties, again moderation is the key now while consuming.

Use red meat processed meat and butter only sparingly. Use re-fined grains, white rice, bread, pasta, potatoes, and sugar containing drinks, sweets and salt sparingly.

Consume healthy fats and oils like olive oil. Extra-virgin olive oil is the best and others like canola, soy, corn, sunflower oils are ok. Use Peanut oil sparingly.

Whole grains, brown rice, whole wheat and oats are preferred.

Have 5 to 7 servings per day of healthy fats like nuts, seeds, olive oil, soy foods and some avocados. Fish is preferred also the best one among is Coldwater fish.

Limit to 2 to 6 servings of fish and seafood per week.

Beans and legumes are rich in magnesium, potassium, soluble fiber, and folic acid.

Non tropical fruits are rich in antioxidants and others.

Bananas, citrus fruits are a natural source of potassium.

Ancillary Food Items not required, but commonly used include:

Addiction: the substances that create euphoria on the first few occasions and subsequently makes to crave for them. Even Sigmund Freud is not the exception for them. This well known person in the field of psychiatry fell victim to cocaine while curiously trying to know it's addiction capabilities. He had to work so hard to get back to himself from its destruction.

Caffeine beverages

Do not contain any essential nutrients. The human body does not require caffeine, but we do use plenty of it. Some people are almost dependent on it on a daily basis to function, and by habit.

Suddenly stopping caffeine intake, can cause headaches, lack of concentration, difficult mood, and may not be able to perform at work, and manage their job efficiently.

Do we certainly need caffeine on a daily basis?

The answer is no. It could help to some extent as a headache medication as needed. People use it to stay awake, which is also a manufactured symptom due to their erratic sleeping habits, hectic schedules or not paying proper attention to the sleeping times?.

To recover from sleep deprivation one needs to sleep. To stay awake or to finish the job, people are opting for caffeinated beverages or other stimulants so that they can get away with the deprived sleep portion from the brain.

Overall, it's not a dangerous medication or substance as long as it is used in limited proportions, as long as a person tolerates with no heart rhythm issues like tachycardia, or stomach issues like ulcers which can get worse with caffeine.

If no other medical condition makes them vulnerable with caffeine, limited intake of caffeine is okay to continue. Try to drink caffeine intake by midday. And It is recommended that way for most people who prefer to sleep at regular hours by 10 PM.

If someone who works the night shift and tries to stay awake by drinking caffeinated beverages, they should stay away from caffeine during daytime that which they assign for sleep.

Some of the beverages with caffeine content in milligrams per cup:

Brewed coffee -- 100-150 mg/cup
Instant coffee--- 85-100 mg/cup.
Tea ---- 60-75 mg/cup.
Cola 40-60 mg/cup.

Decaffeinated means not free of caffeine. It still contains up to 1/5 of the caffeine of regular coffee.

The over-the-counter medications that people use for headaches have a variable amount of up to or more than 100 mg of caffeine per tablet.

Alcohol beverages

F.Scott Fitzgerald a famous American author had been an alcoholic since his college days, and became notorious during the 1920s for his heavy drinking, leaving him in poor health by the late 1930s. Fitzgerald died at age 44.

(Francis Scott Key Fitzgerald (September 24, 1896 – December 21, 1940) was an American author of novels and short stories, whose works are the paradigm writings of the Jazz Age, a term he coined himself. He is widely regarded as one of the greatest American writers of the 20th century. Fitzgerald is considered a member of the "Lost Generation" of the 1920s. He finished four novels: This Side of paradise, The Beautiful and damned, his most famous, The Great Gatsby and Tender is the Night. A fifth, unfinished novel, "The Love of the Last Tycoon", was published posthumously. Fitzgerald also wrote many short stories that treat themes of youth and promise along with despair and age.**)**

Despite food plate/food pyramid recommend alcohol as optional with discretion, I do believe alcohol is not part of the body or brain and is not a food item either. In all possible ways, it should be avoided. People who claim to drink some wine for health purposes should be extremely careful not to exceed the limits and try not to do it into a habit.

In fact, alcohol is the number one non-substance food item causing harm to the users and to others in all possible ways as per the 'drug harms report" in UK a multi-criteria decision analysis study by David Nutt a British psychiatrist and a neuro psycho pharmacologist. Next to that were heroin, crack cocaine, methamphetamines, cocaine, tobacco, amphetamines, marijuana and others. In November 2010, Nutt published in *The Lancet*, co-authored with Les King and Lawrence Phillips on behalf of Independent Scientific Committee on drugs which he founded.

Meanwhile for health purposes if people prefer to drink and if having no contraindications to drink, It is recommended that an average built male is permitted to have 1-2 beers per day with a low alcohol content. Whereas with females it recommended having one beer per each 1-2 days being that it metabolizes slowly in their liver.

But be careful with the medications that you are on. If any interferes with your alcohol, and make sure with your physician.

If you are trying different alcoholic beverages containing different proportions of alcohol by percentage, be prudent to assess and limit the intake should match 1 or 2 beers of total alcohol content per that day.

Certain people with the migraine headaches who want to have some alcoholic beverage during parties and occasions. If they cannot tolerate any other drinks they can try Vodka in a small amount, somehow it is well tolerated in most migraine patients without causing any acute headache.

People with any other brain or psychiatric condition should consult their physician regarding alcohol intake and interactions with medications or contributes to any deterioration or derailment of the neurological status.

Knowing its harmful effects and still it may be useful for some cardiac health, essential tremor like issues but not advised to gravitate towards it.

Shakespeare on alcohol : "It provokes the desire, but it takes away the performance."

Drunkenness is the failure of a man to control his thoughts **–David Grayson.**

There is a link with alcohol abuse and genetics.
There is four times more risk in children of alcoholics that become alcoholics or becoming depressed. Sons effected more than daughters.
Around 1 out of 10 adults are alcohol dependent.
Alcohol is known to reduce the life span as much as 10 years
Females absorb alcohol faster, and it quickly reaches peak blood levels.

Marijuana

Today, marijuana is more popular topic probably replacing the tobacco as used in both recreational and legal form. At this point, some people using marijuana medically for pain relief as seen in use by chronic pain and cancer pain patients. Meanwhile, widely available on streets for recreational purposes, especially being younger generations are overdosing on marijuana with unwanted side effects. As per current census it has only limited purpose in pain management. There is a no general purpose for either daily or routine use just like the case of tobacco.

Overdosing may cause issues with the worsening of depression that we see quite commonly with patients in the hospital. They come back either with the severe decompensation of the depression, panic reactions or impairment of judgment and altered mental state.

We do see some patients complaining dizziness, headaches, and blood pressure issues. Still the long-term negative side effects of this regular use of marijuana is not known regarding any cancer risk or other factors. A lot of research is ongoing. Recent reports show that close to 50% of Americans wanted to see marijuana legalized.

Marijuana causes "Amotivational syndrome" in long-term users meaning loss of desire to function.

Tobacco smoking
Albert Einstein was a heavy smoker.

It is advised to stay away from it. If still smoking, please quit as soon as possible using your willpower. Please see it's harmful effects to you, to the loved one's around you and for the society.

There is no correlation between gender and either attempts to give up cigarettes or the success rate for quitting smoking. The ability to quit depends on the desire to give up the addiction, and how comfortable the person believes the process will be.

It is found that nicotine in tobacco helps Alzheimer's Disease and memory to some extent? But due to the health hazards of smoking every one should stay away from tobacco products. Not every one that smokes get every side effect of it. Who gets what? is not predictable. It curbs the body in its own way over time. It gets to cosmetic effects of blue puffers and pink blotters. Face becomes rough the voice becomes course. Effects are the same of any tobacco product.

Unusual complaints and symptoms with common daily foods

Food allergies : Everybody knows which foods they are allergic to and also if they become allergic to any new food they should avoid it too.

Gluten sensitivity, lactose intolerance and other food related sensitivities are not a matter of this book.

While "Replenish" is limited to briefings on diet regarding brain and mind needs, I present a few unusual symptoms. If anybody is facing them please contact your doctor.

Salt intake

Should be limited and as an as needed basis with one's health conditions.

Nobody needs too much salt unless someone is losing it in excess due to heavy sweating like athletes or people that work under the sun a lot. If anybody is craving for salt, please see your doctor eliminate an Adrenal gland problem like Addison's disease or other medical causes. Patients will have unusual craving for highly salty foods and consume them in large quantities to satisfy their craving.

Eating in moderation is most important. For most of us, we eat than we need, consuming more calories. But if someone is having a **fear of eating** and after the psychiatric causes are eliminated including anorexia nervosa like issues, one should be evaluated to rule out any GI track issues. Mesenteric ischemia causes particular pain in the epigastric region, pain at around the umbilicus that begins shortly after eating. Symptoms usually start half an hour to one hour after eating and can last a few hours. This makes people develop fear of eating or aversion for foods. They start losing weight. It is recommend to pursue further evaluation and management. If they are smokers they should stop soon.

If anybody keeps **getting headaches after a protein rich meal**, consider ornithine transcarbamylase deficiency. This typically occurs after eating a protein rich meal, (usually in childhood) as migraines. Some nausea, vomiting, lethargy and confusion can be associated with these headaches. This headache can be extremely severe. With this particular symptom remember what protein rich meal ate, then necessary testing can be done and treatments are available including limiting the dietary protein.

If somebody get headaches with palpitations and sweating during urination, it may be due to a tumor of the urinary bladder that secretes high catecholamine's called pheochromocytoma. This can cause high blood pressure too.

If the headaches are happening during an orgasm, most of them are truly benign and will go away in few months. They may not recur in few years. But initially leaking aneurysms, bleeding in the brain should be ruled out. If all the work up is negative, nothing to worry about.

We all recommend laughing every day. Everybody thinks that laughing is a sign of good health, a sign of happiness, good mood and keeps us healthy. However, if anybody is **laughing at inappropriate times** all the time or frequently, psychiatric conditions should be ruled out. The possibility of brain diseases like pseudo-bulbar palsy and the progressive supra-nuclear policy should be considered and evaluated. This is due to disintegration, atrophy (shrinking)of parts of the brain due to various yet unknown reasons. But diseases like multiple sclerosis, strokes and Lou Gehrig's Disease can cause emotional lability and inappropriate laughing or even crying. Doctors can further evaluate but still not many treatments available yet. There are few medications that are available as of today. They can at least help to some extent to cut down the emotional lability.

Distaste for smoking cigarettes: we do recommend no smoking. But if any smoker notices sudden loss of taste for cigarettes consider acute viral hepatitis of any type, and can be the reason for the distaste for tobacco.

Pain with Alcohol : consumption in moderation is only optional. I do not recommend any alcohol consumption. Our human body naturally does not need alcohol inside. If anyone gets pain after drinking alcohol as a new symptom, they are advised to see their doctor to rule out cancer called Hodgkin's lymphoma. Many other head, neck, throat cancers, female cancers(breast, uterus, cervical) and bladder cancers can cause this uncommon symptom. Pancreatitis can cause similar complaints. This can proceed months or even years before the diagnosis of cancer is made. Treatment includes, avoiding alcohol and consulting your physician for further management.

A Lot of people like to chew ice or eat large amounts of ice with the beverages: if they are eating to the extent of craving for ice may be having iron deficiency that causes anemia because of various causes of blood loss, including monthly menstrual loss in females. Treating the iron loss and anemia will treat the craving for ice.

Craving for water: we all recommend everybody should drink plenty of water or an adequate amount based on health condition. People with congestive heart failure, liver failure, renal failure and other conditions may need to limit the fluid intake based on your doctor's recommendations. Meanwhile, if anybody is having an intense thirst and craving to consume too much water consider seeing your doctor rule out a disease called diabetes insipidus. This is different from diabetes type I and type II, which are due to insulin deficiency. This is because of central(Brain) or kidney related difficulties with the lack of a hormone called vasopressin in the brain or due to the resistance to vasopressin in the kidneys which makes it not to function properly. This causes enhanced water loss from the kidneys and causes craving for water to replenish. Please see your doctor because many people who have some psychiatric problems or if on some medications can also get into this problem.

Tongue: the most vital organ, to taste, chew, and swallow. It is also the main organ for the articulation of the speech. Meanwhile, if getting pain in the tongue while chewing food, please consider seeing your doctor rule out problems with any poor blood supply to the tongue, due to difficulties with the arteries called atherosclerosis or inflamed arteries called temporal Arteritis. Tongue cancers can be a reason.

Uncommon Tolerances

Lot of pain issues are based on their tolerance, conditioning, cultural, and emotional issues around us.

There are extremes of it and can lead to consequences. Be aware of both hyperalgesia and hypoalgesia. (more sensitive and less sensitive to pain.)

I saw two patients within two days having these extremes.

One morning in the urgent care area, a construction worker in his 20's was brought in with his finger tip chopped and bleeding. The patient did not express any pain. The staff put him in a room, and while making him ready for cauterization to stop the bleeding, he refused any pain medicine, local anesthesia or nerve block. I cauterized his finger with an electric needle. It gave a burning smell, and every body came to look at. This person was calm, quite, and did not show any feelings of discomfort. He came every alternate day for a check up but never asked for pain medication or even complained of pain.

Two days later one 21 year old came in with her boyfriend, crying, screaming ,jumping around in pain. She had a cut on her finger tip while chopping vegetables in the kitchen. Her boyfriend was consoling her and she continued crying.

I went to look at the cut I was surprised. It was just like a razor cut, an extremely tiny superficial laceration on the tip of the finger that did not need any stitches or pain Meds .just Holding pressure and even a band-aid would make it. I discharged her with no concerns.

Both are so extreme examples of pain 'tolerance and intolerance' with a mix of reality, cultural and emotional issues blended.

Part Three

Meditation Techniques & Guidelines

Frustration is common in any activity, occupation or career. Try to relax and take reasonable steps to alleviate it, and come back to your work or practice again. Remember "Moderation" is the Key.

Only when frustration left unattended will turn into laziness, and the target gets ignored.

"Our greatest glory is in never falling but in rising every time we fall" —Confucius

Visualize your changes with imagination.

Meditation

If you are totally new to meditation, the following brief words will explain about this good, better, best and perfect friend.

Meditation is nothing more than having your thoughts fixed on what you want. Your mind will make an ultimatum to your brain to prepare well. That makes it, convey the proper signals back to your mind and body to help recover better and more quickly. You will regain a previous level of functioning as much as possible and also gives you the pleasure of meditation as the joy of the soul. Your joy will reflect on your face, in your words and your acts. That is the power and purpose of daily meditation practice.

The second friend, balanced Diet is extremely essential in the process of recovery. The road to recovery can be smoothened further with ideal dietary practices.

Meditation Techniques

Sit down or recline comfortably.

It is ok to sit down in any comfortable position or to lie down comfortably.

A Few recommendations:

If you cannot get into the 'sit down in classic meditation posture' due to your health condition, or joint issues, then sit down in any comfortable position.

If you choose to lay down, do so comfortably. Either support your head against the headboard of the bed or on a pillow with your arms resting on your chest as in a sleeping position.

Slowly relax your muscles, take a deep breath. Hold it for as long as you can. Make sure your health condition permits this. Holding your breath may not be a good idea or may not be suitable for persons with congestive heart failure, COPD, asthma or other limitations.

You must be more alive and alert in the state of meditation.

Release the breath and take one or two normal breaths.

Again, take a deep breath and hold as long as can. This raises the concentration ability, and calms down the mind to keep it in place by slightly rising your blood concentration of CO_2 (carbon dioxide). Anyone with any medical conditions with limits should not hold their breath, but take normal breaths and continue meditation exercises.

Typically, meditating people concentrate by closing their eyes, but can also focus by looking between the eyes or the area above the nose and between eyebrows, which is called Glabella.

If you cannot do that, there are three other ways to focus.

Sit down in the quiet place while meditating, and listen to the faint pulsating sound in your ears.

If you cannot do that, try to concentrate and listen to your own heart beat while you are taking your breath and releasing it.

If you cannot do that, try to imagine a bright spot with your eyes closed and concentrate on it.

Once you practice and are able to endure it like this, **slowly turn your mind into a goal oriented exercise.**

If your mind wanders for a while, let it be. There is no need to sit down just in one particular meditation posture. **Remember that meditation is a brain exercise, not a body exercise at this point.** People with disabilities, stroke and other neurological conditions, degenerative arthritis, even younger people with the sports injuries and many other issues, cannot maintain a sitting posture in an uncomfortable way. That can destroy the whole concept of the brain training and meditation. Please feel free to find a comfortable spot to do your meditation, rather than one exact meditation posture.

Start slowly taking a deep breath and remain as much and as long as you can.

Slowly your mind releases its hold on negative thoughts and lets it dive deeper, creating rapport with your subconscious mind. Now, both the conscious and subconscious minds are bound together. You can control your mind with your willpower as they are running in harmony.

Exhale slowly.
Recall your goals once again.
Take another deep breath, hold and release.
Slowly your mind will come back to its place.
Do subconscious conversation about your goals.
Continue this for 30 minutes to an hour on a daily basis. Again, the individualized practice guidelines will help further regarding the meditation.

"To climb steep hills requires slow face at first" Shakespeare

Look back and reflect on changes every day before you start your next meditation session. It is like walking on a spiral staircase. You feel like you are still there, but you are going up. In the same way at the beginning, you do not see the results in the geometric proportion. After each day of determination and practice, subconsciously you are making progress and it will show up as a permanent change later. As long as you do not give up, it will be the winner at the end.

Discover the power inside. Unlock and determine the pursuit to be happy and successful. Don't go back in time, think only forward and see what could change. Don't let your mood, and emotions hold you back.

Ask yourself consciously daily in the morning and a few more times during the day:

What is on my mind?
How does my body feel?
What are my goals for today?
How do I feel overall?

This self-inquiry slowly will become a day to day planner.

This will remind of your own state of mind, and will avoid drifting towards worries and negative thoughts, It keeps you goal oriented.

"We are still masters of our own fate. We are still captains of our own souls". —Winston Churchill.

Nobody can help you better than yourself if you fall in the trap of worries vicious cycle. Your dear ones, family, parents and friends can only help to some extent as much as they can. Nobody can do utmost good than yourself. Nobody can intrude into your mind and transform it. Medications and therapies all help to some extent, but only with your conscious effort added to them. If you do not come in harmony with your mind and cannot act in synergy, you cannot stop worries. Finally, you will end up where you are now, going back and forth with rumination. If you are wishing a lifetime change and you want to retain the change, your efforts are most important.

"Twenty years from now you will be more disappointed by the things that you did not do than by the ones you did. So throw off the bowlines. sail away from the safe harbor. Catch the trade winds in your sails. Explore, dream, discovery of challenge, and the joy of growth". —Mark Twain.

Also Remember:

Life - so much to do and not to give up.
Rule your own domain with good control.
You get nothing by sitting in the dark.
You cannot see the light while worrying about the dark.
Be happy, live for today, because yesterday is over, tomorrow do not know about, but expect tomorrow to be the best.
Remain energetic all the time.
Tell yourself that searching for a road in the darkness is boring.
Winning is Yin-Yang always, but trying is not boring. Frustration will make only cause you to fall off more.
Do things that you fear the most one by one - until you see no fear.
Remember that winning is not secure and winners can always lose too.
Do things the best way that you can.

Note

For further reading on self-help Meditation and Rebuilding ourselves topics, refer to " Reveal - Let-It-Go"

Part Four

Individualized diet and meditation session guidelines for each illness – Practice on a daily basis.

Practice daily without giving-up, with the same vigor every day.

Moderation and flexibility are the keys for success in your diet and meditation practices.

Don't ruminate on your illness, but steadfastly practice for improving results.

Your goal is not to worry, but to overcome the issues.

Foggy Brain
Depression
Anxiety
ADD/ADHD
Fibromyalgia

Foggy Brain

Children do not have this without known reasons. If no explanation is identified they will get treated as ADD (Attention Deficit Disorder) or other conditions. Foggy Brain is more prevalent in adults, only slightly more prevalent in females than males, and slightly more prevalent in people with psychiatric concerns and fibromyalgia, than medical illness. It is not the mild cognitive dysfunction of the Alzheimer's type dementia. It is a common complaint of people with fibromyalgia, depression, underlying dysthymia, PTSD, poor sleep, insomnia. Physical ailments not properly treated people with less exposure to sunlight or a deficiency in vitamins or micro nutrients can behave similarly. Fluctuating blood sugars and blood pressures can cause similar symptoms too. It can be chronic and impact lives like pain or fatigue. People can become obsessed with this and ask themselves and others, why they always feel foggy, sluggish, and miserable and cannot feel normal.

Foggy Symptoms:

One feels like wanting to get an electric shock to the brain to charge it or jump-start it.

Symptoms of brain fog can range from mild to severe. They often vary from day to day, and not everyone has all of them. Symptoms include:

difficulty recalling known words, use of incorrect words, or being slow to recall names.

Other symptoms include:

Forgetfulness, the inability to remember what has been read or heard.

Not recognizing familiar surroundings, easily becoming lost, having trouble recalling where things are.

Inability to pay attention to more than one thing, forgetfulness of the original task when distracted.

Trouble processing information, easily distracted.

Difficulty remembering sequences, transposing numbers, trouble remembering numbers.

Feels gloomy all the time, like on a rainy, foggy, cold winter day.

Treatment/Remedies:

Treat pain, insomnia, and feelings of depression and dysthymia.

EXPOSE YOURSELF TO THE SUN DAILY.

Some people do not go out of the house. Those who stay indoors suffer from foggy brain more. Stay in front of the bright light for 15 to 30 minutes every day in the morning.

Anyone with brain fog should consider looking at the sun during the middle of the day briefly, but repeatedly, and have exposure to the sun during the middle of the day as well as in the morning. More sunlight is good to get rid of fatigue, some pain and depression. With sun exposure, the foggy brain becomes brightened -up.

You may feel like transient teaser to your eyes with sudden direct Sun exposure. But there is no risk with only one bit of exposure each time. Do it repeatedly 10 times each day and during the middle of the day. If this is not beneficial, daily exposure to the sun for 30/45 minutes in the morning by sitting directly under the sun or walking in the morning.

You can try daily multivitamin and develop a healthy diet, avoiding excessive meat consumption that makes you sluggish and foggy too. Drink a good amount of fluids and non-sugar, non-stimulating beverages. Some of these good foods are fruits & vegetables, carbohydrates - not refined sugars. fish (Omega-3), Canola or other oils with Omega-3, and eggs. There are people using energy shots and excessive coffee and stimulants. Make sure your health condition permits them and does not cause any side effects with energy drinks. The use of energy drinks should be strongly discouraged.

Mood Disorders

Future for Depression treatments

Strategic deep brain stimulation of specific brain areas is getting evaluated and shows some promise not only for treatment resistant depression, but also for anxiety.

Many new pharmaceutical agents are in the pipeline that will soon be available in the market with hopes of greater benefits to treat depression.

Addressing the social issues, personal triggers are most relevant to address on a continuous basis. The medications are generally useful for endogenous depression. This comes with deficiency or lack of neuro hormones like serotonin and are also helped by medications that balance those neurotransmitters. Other type of depression needs to be addressed with many different modes of therapies.

ADD/ADHD

Adult ADD is very tricky for both the person and for the physician to diagnose.

It manifests with no hyperactivity, but with a sense of inner restlessness, resulting infrequent job changes, inability to work, disorganized work, poor self-esteem, undertaking of risky behaviors, clashes with authorities, frequent injuries, easy frustration, childish behavior and under achievement.

If you have some of these features your physician can evaluate and eliminate other possible causes

Future treatments for ADD/ADHD

Although there is no immediate cure, a new understanding of Attention Deficit Disorder and ADHD may be forthcoming. This will ultimately result in improving the personal fulfillment and productivity of people with ADHD. New, non-stimulant medications are on their way, albeit slowly.

Additional research is ongoing to determine the long-term outcome.

One by one, studies are conducted by scientists and they are beginning to understand the biological nature of attention disorders. New research is allowing them to better understand the inner workings of the brain and to develop new medications and evaluate different forms of treatment.

ADD/ADHD

Short-term prognosis

In about 15% of preschool children, there is a particular concern about ADHD, with 5% associated with children during the elementary school years.

Long-term prognosis

Many children and adolescents do not outgrow ADHD.

Associated symptoms and aggressive behavior can bring a poor, long-term prognosis.

ADHD may manifest in different ways in the adult as compared to the child.

Depression/Anxiety/ADD/ADHD (trio)

Diet Mind

It is not your fault. In most cases, the above issues are either familial, endogenous, environmental or circumstances coupled with daily life stressors are co-existing..

Eliminating the co-existing things causing the trio or any one of them is the diet mind.

Look inward and log the reasons for your depression, anxiety, and attention deficit disorder (ADD).

Write down the times (such as morning, evening, winter, fall) that make you more vulnerable. In females, the menstrual cycle may make them more vulnerable during that time.

Write down all of the situations that make you feel depressed, anxious, show a lack of motivation, attention and concentration.

Learn to say "No". More than 25% of the time, especially in the younger population, it is one of the precipitants. You do not want to do something, but you cannot say "No" due to peer pressure and other stressors. That causes internal conflict, restlessness, worry, rumination and unnecessary, anticipated anxiety and depression.

Face the fear from within until you extinguish it - day by day.

Read this Daily

Life is long, and there is much more to do.

Life has endless possibilities and pleasures if you are goal oriented.

Vigor and energy can only enhance the brain function.

Do everything that makes you anxious, one thing at a time.

Think about everything that makes depressed, one thing at a time.

Face everything that makes you depressed or anxious in a challenging way.

Face the feelings with effort and do not run away from the situation.

As a child, you did the same. You fell down and stood up again and again until you learned to walk perfectly.

You can fall down and stand up from depression and anxiety until you are no longer depressed or anxious.

Life is short. There is only enough time to be happy, and to enjoy the pleasures, so do not lose time for sadness and unrest.

Accept the depression and anxiety as just another life experience to compare to and learn from it.

Recall some famous people who went through similar stages like Charles Darwin, Sigmund Freud, and JK Rowling.

Stay away from any stimulants, drugs.

Tobacco makes feel better now, but makes you feel worse later.

When anticipatory anxiety comes on, tell yourself to postpone it until the actual event occurs.

When anxiety prevails during the act or event, let it ride with you rather than you trying to hide it. Let it pass through like – just as you do not feel the rain when walking in the rain.

Try not to create more ripples in the mind. React to anxiety/depression by just ignoring it.

Meditation is perfect for ADD/ADHD, anxiety and depression.

If you cannot concentrate and meditate on anything in particular, just think of someone that you like most, or something that you like most, creating brain activity that takes you away from your current activity.

Take brief siestas/naps, if possible just to calm your brain and mind.

Limit your intake to 1 or 2 cups of regular coffee or tea if cannot stop altogether.

Limit your intake to 1 beer per day or alternate one beer and an approximate alcoholic beverage if cannot stay away from it completely. You should stay far away from any mind altering drugs, alcohol and non-prescription stimulants.

Adult ADD/ADHD needs a lot of self-questioning. With Biofeedback, learn to speak only as needed. You can get the same results from therapies and psychological counseling.

People with depression, anxiety, and ADD get a lot of sleep issues and body aches, which can lead to fibromyalgia or migraines, chronic sleep difficulties, insomnia and fits.

Your goal is not to get those. You want to be productive and enjoy the pleasures of life.

Do not skip doses of your prescription medicines and/or counseling appointments.

Self- counseling is studying your mind and taking away the mental blocks and obstacles that cause or aggravate your depression, anxiety, and ADD and helps to eliminate them effectively.

Despite good potential, a lot of patients with ADD/ADHD, anxiety and depression miss opportunities.

They change jobs frequently, do not reach their potential and will have recurring troubles with higher authorities at their workplace.

Self-counseling and self words used in situations where 'you need them more than they want you' and "you want to become indispensable by showing your talent and skills" will help.

A positive approach and progress at work puts your trio on shelf. Day by day, will take good results at work, at home and personally.

Brain Diet

ADD/ADHD

Take any medication that has been prescribed regularly.

Maintain regular hours for sleep. Get enough sleep - at least seven to eight hours each night if are not a short sleeper.

Do regular exercise at least 20 to 30 minutes on most days of the week.

Do meditation calming your mind. Use deep-breathing techniques to help with anxiety and anger.

Relaxation training and meditation will help to increase focus and concentration, as well as lower distractions.

Eliminate items from the diet that you think are causing difficulties with attention, anger, and being distracted.

Find with self-experimentation, the foods that help to soothe your mind and adhere to them in a regular fashion.

If have any food allergies or allergies to additives, they need to be avoided. You will see only by trying and having self-experiences.

It is reasonable to avoid these substances such as artificial colors, mostly red and yellow.

Avoid food additives such as aspartame, MSG (monosodium glutamate), and nitrites. Some studies have linked hyperactivity to the intake of the preservative sodium benzoate.

Some people do get hyperactive after eating candy or other sugary foods.

Caffeine and ADHD:

Some studies have shown that small amounts of caffeine may help with some ADHD symptoms. However, the side effects of caffeine may outweigh any potential benefit. Most recommend avoiding caffeine as much as possible. Having small amounts usually in the morning and afternoon is ok.

Make any dietary changes slowly over time, but eliminate the foods that are causing ADD/ADHD symptoms quickly.

Overall

Eat a high protein diet that includes beans, eggs, meat, fish and nuts. Eat less of total sugars and fewer simple carbohydrates such as candy, corn syrup, honey, products made from white flour, white rice, and potatoes. Eat more vegetables and fruits, including oranges, citrus, pears, apples, and kiwi.

ADD/Depression/Anxiety Meditation

Try meditation in common sitting position if possible.

Do as Long as can for more than half an hour to one hour per day minimum.

Limit meditation to once or twice a day.

Morning is the best time for meditation.

Sleep time meditation as the next session is useful. The bedtime meditation can be done in sleeping posture. Okay to slip into sleep while doing meditation.

Depression

Tell yourself:

Nobody is the winner.
It is 50/50 chance.
Nobody is a loser.
If you think only about dusk, you cannot appreciate the light.
It is too boring to walk in the dark.

Diet in depression:

Make sure your medications are helping, make sure use them regularly.

Follow a good diet program.

Look good to yourself. It makes a lot of difference in your self-esteem.

When look at yourself in the mirror, you should be asking yourself what is lacking to make you feel depressed. This means your appearance brings more self-esteem and motivation. Stand in front of the mirror alone, calm and quiet and have a brief conversation with yourself. It is like exploring self.

Eat right and eat well. Maintain excellent table manners, especially while dining with others or family members.

Choose your foods carefully.

Even though, there is no specific diet plan for depression, eat regularly, without skipping meals and without overeating.

Avoid snacks and drinking sodas, which are quite often consumed while depressed along with sitting on the couch. Anorexia is also common.

Good Foods

Eat a normal range of proteins, carbohydrates and fats.

Avoid high protein and high calorie food.

Avoid all stimulants other than prescription medications, including coffee, not drinking it more than twice a day by afternoon if prefer.

Expose yourself to sunlight by afternoon every day for 30 minutes to 1 hour.

Take vitamin D and a multivitamin daily, as needed.

Beans and legumes, lean meat like chicken and turkey, low-fat dairy products, nuts and seeds are good. Sea foods and whole grains should be mainly on a daily routine.

Eat whatever feel like on festive occasions and at parties. Stay away from large quantities or habitual use of alcohol.

Anxiety Diet

Work on your anticipatory anxiety first.

Practice Biofeedback, meditation daily.

Avoid Coffee, alcohol and all other stimulants.

A slightly higher protein diet on a daily basis is good.

Avoid pure sugars and snacks.

Eat more fruits.

Because of your anxiety, if have IBS or lack of sleep, drink more fluids, but avoid beverages including coke, diet drinks.

Pay attention to food sensitivities.

Try to eat healthy, balanced meals.

Try to avoid fried foods, choosing fruits like peaches or berries, or nuts like almonds instead.

Fibromyalgia

Take doctors advice and get your medications regularly.

Do not give up on medications by trying them for a short while or small, initial doses.

A lot of medications for fibromyalgia need to be used and tried for a longer run at optimal doses before concluding that particular medication is not for you.

Diet mind

Think of fibromyalgia as a non-life-threatening illness.

It will not do harm to any of your vital organs.

It does not damage your heart, brain, kidneys or any other vital organs.

It is a chronic and painful illness and can be debilitating to muscles and the fascia.

Even knowing this, you will come to the conclusion that it is the still a blessing compared to people with cancers and other serious illnesses.

Maintain strict daily routine.

Good sleep is highly beneficial.

Go to bed at regularly scheduled times, preferably around 10:30 PM., with a wake up time around 6:30 a.m.

Before getting up, stay in bed for 10 minutes trying to meditate, or sit down quietly.

Afterwards, get up out of the bed and stretch all of your muscles, neck, spine, hips, shoulders, elbows and arms.

Walk from room to room, preferably on carpet, on toes and heels, doing this twice.

Go and get a large drink - either a bottle of water or grape or orange juice.

Try not to drink coffee, coke, any caffeinated beverage or alcohol.

Go and get a good hot shower.

Stretch all muscles before you put on your clothes.

Stretch your fingers and wrist and elbow joints. Follow simple stretching exercises.

Now get ready and go to your work as vigorously as possible after a good breakfast.

While at work try to stretch all muscles up to three times a day.

Try to get a siesta or nap, just for 10 minutes during mid-day. You need not go into deep sleep, just try to relax and forget about the world, your surroundings, and about yourself. Say to yourself that you are not there.

Take one day at a time to treat your fibromyalgia.

Stretching never hurts.

Brain diet

Eat regularly and moderately with variety, quality and quantity.

Choose foods that you tolerate well.

Avoid high sugars, caffeinated sodas, diet colas, some vegetables like tomatoes, broccoli, cabbage, and cauliflower.

Avoid caffeine, artificial sweeteners, MSG like substances.

Drink plenty of fluids, eat whole grains as tolerated, and balanced food with meat, protein, fish, egg whites and cereals.

If overweight, try to cut down fatty foods further.

If tolerates taking a daily vitamin with minerals is good.

Get exposure to enough sunlight daily by afternoon. Avoid evening sun.

Get exposure to the morning sun for half an hour to one hour. Melatonin aids in better sleep. If one sleeps well, 50% of their pain is gone the next day. Do meditation if possible in the afternoon or evening.

Use morning time for stretching exercises.

Maintain daily standard sleep times.

Do not sleep at odd times.

If you take a brief nap, limit to half an hour to 45 minutes only.

Prefer standard meditation practice unless not able to sit down

If possible, do this at least two or three times per day.

Diet and Neurological Disorders

Traumatic Brain Injuries
&
Post-Concussion Syndrome

Post concussion syndrome and traumatic brain injuries prove that we are not alone and does not discriminate. Many people from all types of life have had traumatic brain injuries and suffered from their consequences.

Doctors will explain your injuries and the extent of expected recovery. Once all the work-up done, after acute care and recovery therapies take prescribed medicines regularly.

Diet Mind

Many recover fully. Many suffer different consequences.

The people who recovered well still can have minor and subtle memory issues, headaches, seizures as consequences.

People who had serious issues when recovered with lifelong consequences like paralysis, dementia, disabled functions still can Perform better with the constant practice and determination, and by keeping the frustration and depression away.

In the post concussion syndrome, the symptoms of depression, frustration, irritability, short-term memory issues, tinnitus, ringing in the years, light sensitivity, sleep difficulties should improve in the weeks or few months mostly.

The wobbly feeling or any dizziness should improve too.

Take necessary therapies, try to maintain a regular lifestyle, stay away from stimulants, alcohol, and use as needed hypnotic, short-term anxiolytics with your doctor's advice.

Brain Diet

Stay away from food that makes drowsy like high fatty and protein diets.

Go with the low-carb, avoid pure sugars in excess, prefer fresh vegetables, fruits, and juices.

Limit your coffee to morning and afternoon.

Expose to sunlight during daytime.

Maintain normal sleeping hours especially waking up in the morning at the same time daily.

Avoid straining at the toilet, Avoid constipation.

Empty the bladder without waiting until too full.

You can take short-term hypnotic agents, but avoid any habit-forming agents.

Do regular stretching and other exercises.

Do mentally stimulating activity without getting fatigued or getting frustrated. Video games and games like chess can be preferred, including doing puzzles.

Play physically active simple sports avoiding further trauma.

Treat your symptoms as needed with the therapies.

Short-term prognosis

More than 80% of patients with the mild TBI and post concussion syndrome recovered from the neurologic stigmata within six weeks to three months, but older individuals may recover considerably more slowly.

A small percentage - around 15% - have persistent post-concussion syndrome symptoms beyond a year after injury owing to multiple interacting, physiologic and psychological factors.

Long-term prognosis

Most with mild to moderate injury return to work between one and six months. Most of those with severe injuries return to work between six and 12 months and a significant number required up to two years.

Continuing improvements in functioning has been observed inpatients even beyond 1 to 2 years after injury.

TBI has a relatively long course of recovery and greater prognosis for long-term improvement in functional status than do most other neurological disorders.

Lot of help we can get from meditation

Recommended for everyone with the traumatic brain injury.

Many symptoms of easy irritability, sensation of lightheadedness, sensitivity to sound and light, ringing in ears, lack of sleep, concentration all can get better with meditation.

Maintain standard routine sleep times.

Stay away from all stimulants.

Drink plenty of water daily.

When wake up in the morning sit up in the bed and, do meditation briefly for 15 to 20 minutes.

Before coming of the bed sit down another 5to 10 minutes in bed.

Finish your activities of daily living.

If not going to work after breakfast sit down for another 15 to 30 minutes for meditation session.

If possible, do tai chi and balance exercises.

If working, do your routine job related duties.

Expose to sun, natural light intermittently.

Dizziness & Vertigo

Several etiologies included. The diagnosis needs thorough history, examination and necessary testing.

Depending on how long each episode lasts the most common causes are Benign vertigo(BPPV),TIA, Migraine, Vertebrobasilar insufficiency, strokes, labyrinthitis, MS, trauma, Minier's disease and others.

Treatment depends on the correct diagnosis and includes both medical and surgical in some cases.

Several patients needs help from a group of Doctors that cover your PCP, Neurologist or Neurosurgeon, ENT specialist, Balance testing, Gait training, Physical therapist and Others.

In U.S. average 5.5 million patient visits occur to doctor's offices because of dizziness and/or vertigo.

Famous people reported having tinnitus:

Vincent van Gogh: (30 March 1853 – 29 July 1890) was a Dutch post -impressionist painter.

Michelangelo: (6 March 1475 – 18 February 1564), was an Italian Renaissance sculptor, painter, architect, poet, and engineer who exerted an unparalleled influence on the development of western art.

Charles Darwin: (12 February 1809 – 19 April 1882) was an English naturalist.

Ronald Reagan: (February 6, 1911 – June 5, 2004) was the 40th president of United States of America (1981–89).

Howard Hughes : (December 24, 1905 – April 5, 1976) was an American business magnate, investor, aviator, aerospace engineer, filmmaker and philanthropist..

Dizziness/Vertigo, Lightheadedness/Tinnitus

Seek your doctor's advice, needed testing, imaging and treatments to fallow and find out all medical and neurological and psychiatric, ENT causes. Sometimes overmedicating is another reason for your symptoms.

Take all safety measures to prevent falls and other traumas.

Diet Mind

Dizziness/Vertigo, Lightheadedness / Tinnitus can be disabling and can be chronic issues.

Frustration and worry about something else can cause these symptoms worse.

That is why should have proper work-up. If doctors could not find any reason specifically to treat your condition and if still have symptoms, that is the time that want to work on your frustration.

Bio feed back and self counseling saying that you are happy with no stroke, brain tumor and that you are happy with no surgery on your brain is necessary, makes you relieve some of your symptoms.

Attend PT/OT and balance therapies as much as possible to alleviate your symptoms.

Brain can relearn the balance and alleviate dizziness and ringing to some extent but needs self practice.

Use muffling sounds for tinnitus to ignore the ringing.

Just meditate or concentrate only on ringing of the ear or another vibrating sound daily 10 minutes for 3 times a day to improve the tinnitus, dizziness, and vertigo.

Stand at the wall with back support or stand on a firm bed if can for 10 minutes at a time for 3 times a day to improve the dizziness, balance.

Drink plenty of fluids and do not get constipated on a regular basis

Empty the bladder without waiting too long. Full bladder stimulates the autonomic nervous system and makes the symptoms worse.

Nighttime if needs to come out of the bed do it slowly and with good light around.

Take brief naps during the daytime up to 2 times but less than 30 minutes each time.

Meditation, Yoga and Tai chi, acupuncture can help too.

Do other stretching exercises to relax the muscles in and around the head, ears and neck.

Epley Maneuver that trains to treat your vertigo at home is useful too.

Make sure anxiety, allergies, and gluten in food in some cases are not causing these symptoms.

Brain Diet

Low salt diet is good.

Low carbohydrate, low sugar diet is good.

Plenty of fluids is good.

Up to 2 cups of small coffee/ decaffeinated coffee/ 1 coke beverage is reasonable to try, may help dizziness and ease the ringing in ears.

As a stimulant, caffeine can worsen tinnitus, which is a ringing sound in your ear that may accompany vertigo. So try if it helps or worsens and decide to continue or stop.

can try Ginkgo- Biloba.

Go with fruits, nuts, and cereals with minerals and magnesium but less salty. Generally include nuts, seeds, beans and leafy green vegetables.

Avoid citrus fruits or other that irritates your stomach, can provoke nausea and dizziness. Salty Foods also to avoid..

Avoid a high-sodium diet. Sodium-rich Prepared foods include canned soups and vegetables, frozen meals, pretzels, French fries, crackers, tomato sauce, cold cuts, hot dogs, bacon and processed cheese.

Avoid Added Sugars. When consume a sugary food, keep your portion size modest and pair it with other foods, such as whole grains or low-fat milk, to prevent the blood sugar imbalances.

Avoid Migraine Triggers.

If dizzy episodes are associated with migraine headaches, foods that trigger your migraines may also cause vertigo.

Avoid Alcohol unless it helps your tinnitus and dizziness in small amounts.

Overall Diet rich in plant foods, minerals, potassium, magnesium, vitamins, low in sugars and fats, can be more useful for dizziness

Dizziness and vertigo meditation

stay in bed 5 minutes before getting up from sleep in the morning.

Stay another five minutes in a sitting position with the legs hanging on the side of the bed.

Morning is the best for meditation.

Twice a day is recommended.

If possible maintain the posture either in the sitting position either on the ground or chair. The dizziness vertigo spells decrease with the meditation.

Maintain good sleep hygiene practices too.

Epilepsy and seizure disorders

When Seizures or fits happen again and again or at least more than twice, they are called Epilepsy. They are several types like grand mal, absence, partial complex and can be disabling. They endanger the patient's daily routines with restrictions on driving and at work can restrict the capabilities. Also, Most seizure patients suffer from chronic depression. Most seizures do not cause either mental retardation or deterioration of intelligence. This has been proved beyond all doubt by whom achieved extraordinary things in spite of suffering from epilepsy.

Fortunately several medications called Antiepileptic drugs are available. Many new better medications are coming. Electroencephalogram(EEG) with or without video monitoring and Ambulatory EEG are done to diagnose the seizure type so can be treated accurately with proper medications.

Most Seizure patients need imaging of the brain by MRI, ,CT scans. For patients with uncontrolled seizures, new surgical procedures and vagal nerve stimulation procedures are available to control.

With well-controlled seizures on medications, any patient can resume their daily duties with out several restrictions.

The Driving precautions and suggestions are provided either in the local DMV for each state or available on the Internet.

Historical and Famous people with Epilepsy or seizures or spells of a similar nature:

Julius Caesar: (July 100 BC – 15 March 44 BC) was a Roman general, statesman, and notable author of Latin prose.

Alfred Nobel: Noble prize founder.(21 October 1833 – 10 December 1896) was a Swedish chemist, engineer, innovator, and armaments manufacturer. He was the inventor of dynamite. He had febrile seizures in infancy.

Vincent Van Gogh: (30 March 1853 – 29 July 1890) was a Dutch post-impressionist painter. Over 150 physicians have produced nearly 30 different diagnoses for van Gogh's illness. Henri Gastaut's posthumous diagnosis was "temporal lobe epilepsy precipitated by the use of absinthe in the presence of an early limbic lesion". This agrees with that of van Gogh's own doctor, Felix Rey, who prescribed potassium bromide.. That van Gogh's personality closely matches the Geschwind syndrome(A characteristic personality syndrome seen both in the inter-ictal (between seizures) and the ictal (during seizures) states.) is seen as further evidence by some. Not everyone agrees – a recent review by John Hughes concluded that van Gogh did not have epilepsy. He certainly was mentally ill at times and had "fainting fits" after heavy drinking.

Napoleon Bonaparte :(15 August 1769 – 5 May 1821) was a French military and political leader who rose to prominence during the latter stages of the French Revolution and its associated wars in Europe. As Napoleon I, he was Emperor of the French from 1804 to 1815. A paper by William Osler in 1903 stated, "The slow pulse of Napoleon rests upon tradition; it has been suggested that his epilepsy and attacks of apathy may have been associated features in a chronic form of Stokes-Adams disease", which implies the seizures were not epileptic in origin. However, in 2003, John Hughes concluded that Napoleon had both Psychogenic attacks due to stress and epileptic seizures due to chronic uremia from a severe urethral stricture.

Hercules: Greek mythological hero.

Alexander the Great: Alexander III of Macedon (20/21 July 356 – 10/11 June 323 BC), commonly known as Alexander.

Leo Tolstoy:(September 9, 1828 – November 20, 1910) was a Russian writer who primarily wrote novels and short stories. Later in life, he also wrote plays and essays. His writings had a profound impact on such pivotal twentieth-century figures as Mahatma Gandhi and Martin Luther King, Jr. Tolstoy had "Fits of spleen" and anguish attacks. Had seizures while dying of Pneumonia.

Michelangelo: (6 March 1475 – 18 February 1564 was an Italian Renaissance sculptor, painter, architect, poet, and engineer who exerted an unparalleled influence on the development of Western art. Michelangelo had a faint due to working in very hot weather.

Socrates: (469 BC – 399 BC) was a Classical Greek Athenian Philosopher. Credited as one of the founders of Western philosophy. It is speculated that his daimonion was a simple partial seizure and that he had temporal lobe epilepsy.

Leonardo Da Vinci: (April 15, 1452 – May 2, 1519,) was an Italian Renaissance polymath painter, sculptor, architect, musician, mathematician, engineer, inventor, anatomist, geologist, cartographer, botanist, and writer. He had nervous shaking and spasms when furious.

Franklin Delano Roosevelt: (January 30, 1882 – April 12, 1945), also known by his initials, FDR, was the 32nd President of the united States(1933–1945) and a central figure in world events during the mid-20th century, leading the United States during a time of worldwide economic depression and total war. He thought to have complex partial seizures attributable to cerebrovascular disease.

Seizures/Epilepsy and Diet

Make sure no brain tumor or other serious cause exists for your seizures.

See your doctor regularly and take your medications regularly with punctuality.

Lot of the anti seizure medications work only 8- 12 hours and missing few doses is enough to get a breakthrough seizure.

Diet Mind

Despite a worrisome /horrible disease many are well controlled and are functional.

The goal is "seizure free" but not just having fewer seizures.

The goal is getting back to driving and other usual activities that one performs normally.

Lots of seizures will subside by young adult hood.

Lots of seizures become easily controlled over time.

Few unfortunate may need many medications, vagal nerve stimulation and brain surgeries to remove the epileptic areas of the brain.

Maintain healthy, routine life style.

Avoid all triggers like sleep deprivation mainly, stimulants, extreme tiredness, fatigue, and too much mental and physical exhaustion, bright or flashing lights.

Control panic or anxiety, tension or stress.

If any high fever occurs handle immediately.

Meditate relax mentally on a daily basis.

Imagine your self-a everyday life and your goal is to achieve that.

Brain Diet for Seizures

High fat, ketogenic diet is proved to be useful. But causes difficulties with oily stools, smelly, greasy stool and discomfort. Weight gain, raising cholesterol, kidney stones are the other troubles.

Low sugar diet helps.

Most of Calories will be derived from fats such as hot dogs, mayonnaise, and butter, potato chips.

Vegetables such as carrots, broccoli, spinach, and lettuce fall into the unrestricted category,

Take multivitamin a day while on this diet to ensure that one's nutritional needs are met.

The Atkins diet may be an effective alternative for children who have a difficult time complying with the ketogenic diet.

Low carbohydrate and high protein diet are another alternative.

Seizures Meditation

Sleep adequately.

After waking up see whether still feeling groggy because of your nighttime seizure medications.

If you are groggy, do not sit down for meditation.

Go on with your daily morning activities.

When feeling refreshed and vibrant with the nighttime medication effects are over then do meditation and half an hour to one hour is enough.

Lot of seizures are triggered by stress.

Lot of seizure like spells are not seizures.

Concentrate on your stress relief from your meditation.

Meditation should help you to ignore seizure like spells, helps you to ignore the anticipated anxiety for seizures.

Meditation should help you to get the seizures less frequent and easily manageable.

Short-term prognosis

Is great with the management of precipitating/ triggers for seizures.

Once serious causes ruled out, taking the medications regularly and avoiding all the triggers makes the seizure prevention better.

Long-term prognosis

for control of Seizures with the treatment is excellent in most of the generalized seizure types.

The partial seizures experience a higher recurrence rate. Approximately 75% of patients with epilepsy will achieve remission within five years of diagnosis. However those patients who have not achieved remission after five years are less likely to achieve full seizure cessation.

Stroke or Brain attack and TIA

Each year there are 700,000 people (one every 45 seconds) in the United States who suffer a stroke.

These present as sudden loss or difficulty of speech, arm or leg weakness or numbness, transient loss of vision, difficulty of balance and walking.

Advances in Neuroscience and Imaging modalities as MRI/CTA of Brain revolutionized the treatment of stroke in recent years.

With any acute symptoms of stroke or TIA, please call EMS and go to the nearest emergency room for immediate and appropriate care.

Unfortunately, most strokes are painless and happen during sleep, and we have only limited time to act.

But for limited patients in the Time window the medications or catheter procedures with Intra arterial therapy and cerebral angioplasty are useful to prevent brain damage.

Close monitoring and early rehabilitation after acute stroke are vital in patient recovery and long-term outcome to regain their normal activities.

Transient Ischemic attacks For patients with warning strokes called TIA's the ultrasound (carotid duplex and TCD)and imaging tests will tell us accurately who should be treated with Aspirin or other blood thinners and who needs carotid surgery or stent placements to prevent future strokes. patients with non-critical narrowing of carotid blood vessels that supply to brain, need regular interval fallow-up to detect the progression of the disease and correct it as needed.

Disease Modifiers Also controlling Diabetes, cholesterol, high blood pressure, changing life style like avoiding smoking, alcohol and illicit drugs and performing regular exercises play a major role in preventing future strokes.

Future For Unfortunate Stroke victims for whom above therapies and rehabilitation are not sufficient to recover adequately, we hope a new modality of treatment called Trancranial magnetic stimulation will be available. These patients may benefit further to recover their damaged brain function by neuroplasticity. It is widely used already in Europe.

Summer risks for stoke

No one over the age of 50, not even a lifelong athlete in seemingly excellent health are free from the risk of stroke. However, there are some preventive measures believed to limit the recurrence and the extent of damages.

With people living longer and the modern era of pre-made and pre-packaged foods, the rate of strokes has increased. Over the last several decades, stroke prevention measures have not changed much, but more awareness about stroke and its devastating nature are getting wider publicity.

"The most important part of stroke prevention is what is known as primary prevention. Other than genetically predisposing components, the way we eat, live and care for our bodies are the primary ways we can impact our risk. Other than your primary care physician, the people who may be most important in stroke prevention are parents, and how they supervise what their children eat, help develop dietary habits, choose active daily lifestyles and make a conscious effort to keep body and mind healthy."

Primary Stroke Prevention Measures

who wish to impact their risk of stroke

Eat a healthy diet. Have enough daily proportions of protein, fat, carbohydrates, nutrients, vitamins and minerals that do not exceed the total calorie need for the individual's body mass index. This will avoid excessive accumulation of body fat and diet induced obesity.

Get enough regular exercise to increase endurance and burn or use excess calories.

Maintain a healthy mind with particular consideration to controlling stress, exhaustion and emotions.

Get enough sleep without indulging in excess laziness of body and mind.

Avoid alcohol, smoking and other stimulants.

"Despite all these efforts, if medical issues arise such as high blood pressure, Diabetes, high cholesterol or absorption issues that cause vitamin deficiencies get treatment for the conditions and monitor it regularly.

Seasonal Precautions

Surprisingly, seasonal activities sometime impact the risk of stroke.

Summer: "The elderly are more at risk of stroke during the summer due to dehydration either because of inadequate fluid intake or medications that cause impaired sweating and heat exhaustion with outdoor activity. Stay well hydrated and be aware of medications and their side effects."

Holidays. "Inadequate intake of water and excessive consumption of alcohol that can lead to related complications including hemorrhagic and infraction strokes is worth mentioning. Limit alcohol intake to one glass of wine or beer every other day for females due to a slower liver metabolism and one glass of wine or beer every day for males."

Nutritional Supplements

"While many people take numerous dietary supplements, there is no miracle supplement pill as of yet. "Supplements that contain B6, B12, and folate as a combination pill and MVI may be taken daily. Ask your physician to test for any specific vitamin deficiencies. People at high risk for stroke may need to have their homocysteine, methionine or B12, and folate levels checked too. Some supplements such as fish oils and garlic were noted to have good effects on blood vessels."

Preventive Screening Tests

"Have your doctor review your history, examination and evaluate your risk factors such as your lipid profile, blood pressure, blood sugar, thyroid, and homocysteine levels. If you are found to be in a high-risk group, your doctor may refer you for further screening. There are additional screenings that can be done should your physician find it necessary.

"In summary, the most effective way to reduce your risk of stroke is to lead a healthy lifestyle and get regular checkups with your primary care physician."

Examples of few Notables who suffered from strokes

Alfred Bernhard Nobel :(21 October 1833 – 10 December 1896) was a Swedish chemist, engineer, innovator, and armaments manufacturer. He was the inventor of dynamite. Alfred Nobel died of bleeding in the brain (cerebral hemorrhage) in 1896.

This is not the stroke due to the blocked or stenotic blood vessels which is more common than bleeding in the brain. But both can cause similar consequences.

Winston Churchill

The British statesman and prime minister had a stroke in 1949 and another in 1953. He remained active after his strokes and was active in Parliament until 1959. It was after his strokes that he supervised the development of the British hydrogen bomb as well as the publication of his multi-volume History of the English Speaking People in the late 1950s.

Louis Pasteur

The man responsible for the vaccines for anthrax and rabies was permanently paralyzed on the left side by a stroke in 1868. Almost all of his immunology research was completed after his stroke.

Dwight D. Eisenhower :Eisenhower, a general and United States president, had a stroke in 1955 from which he recovered quickly. He was elected to a second term in 1956 and completed an entire second presidency. He remained active after he retired, and authored several books.

Stroke/TIA

Stroke: Most people recover well/ mostly due to brain plasticity.

The strategically located strokes may take longer time and may be difficult to recover to the full extent of the previous level of function.

The residual deficits may disable the person. The person who suffered stroke should not neglect any mode of therapy that will let the brain recover faster.

Stroke precautions: Patients with medical problems like hypertension, diabetes, high cholesterol, obstructive sleep apnea, Obesity, family history of strokes will need particular attention to treat those conditions called secondary stroke prevention. Controlling well your medical conditions will help to eliminate the higher risk of stroke.

Elderly: With or without stroke risk are prone to have strokes if they become dehydrated, nutritionally debilitated, inactive, exposed to some medications, especially in summer with different ways of dehydration.

Once all the necessary medical, environmental precautions were taken fallowing good dietary habits staying away from smoking tobacco, stimulants, heavy coffee or other self-injuring behaviors will help further.

The Good diet plate will help further preventing strokes and longevity with physical and mental happiness.

Diet Plate for Stroke/TIA patients

Prefer mostly vegetarian, white meat, limit calories to 2000 calorie /day.

Adequate fluids around 2 liters per day. If a person got renal or Heart failure issues, take the amount of fluid that is allowed as per doctors advice.

If not allergic, 2 cups of regular milk are good per day.

Ok with 1-2 small cups of regular /decaf coffee/tea before 4PM any time.

Egg white with no yolk good even on a daily basis.

Limit meat including Red or white to 2 times/week. Still keep the total calories within 2000 calories/day.

Daily walking or other types of activity as much as you can or Up to 30-45 minutes /day.

Go to sleep regularly and wake up at regular time every day including weekends.

when wake up stay in bed for 10 minutes and try to meditate consciously. It is ok if slip into REM sleep during that 10 minutes, it can make you restored, refreshed and can tune the autonomic nervous system.

start your day calm and quiet. Give preference to intellectual or other thinking process-related issues in the morning.

Start your daily tasks that involves physical /manual demand.

Continue to keep well hydrated during the day.

Maintain inner calmness, self-meditating efforts while working and while taking breaks.

You will see new energy day by day even by the end of the day.

If possible middle of the day break try to take 10-minute meditation nap. Need not meditate, but sit down quite and comfortably even in parked garage inside the car with emptiness of your mind. If can take a nap, it will refresh to 10 times more active for afternoon work.

Stroke Diet Plate

Whatever you do, watch for low salt foods. Low Sodium intake is good not only for stroke prevention but to overall health and stroke recovery.

Eat foods that do not cause or prevent constipation. Straining with constipation will adversely affect the stroke patients by increasing intracranial pressure each time that they strain.

Prefer

Grains: Make sure at least half of your choices from this group come from whole grains.

Vegetables: Choose often-nutrient rich dark green and orange vegetables and remember to eat regularly dried beans and peas.

Fruits: Eat a variety of fresh, frozen or dried fruits each day.

Protein: Choose low-fat or lean meats, poultry; and remember to vary your choices with more beans, peas, nuts, seeds and fish sources. In terms of fats, make most of your fat sources from fish, nuts and vegetable oils. Limit fat sources from butter, margarine, shortening or lard.

Dairy: Choose low-fat or fat-free dairy foods, or a variety of non-dairy calcium-rich foods each day.

Choose foods high in fiber

As part of a heart-healthy diet, fiber can reduce cholesterol and your overall risk for cardio, Cerebro vascular disease. Dietary fiber is part of plants that body cannot digest. As it passes through your body, it affects the way your body digests food and absorbs nutrients. How much fiber? you eat affects not only your cholesterol level and risk for stroke, but may have other health benefits: helps control blood sugar, promotes regularity, prevents gastrointestinal disease and helps in weight management.

Most of us fall short of the recommended daily fiber guidelines of 21 -38 grams per day. Too much fiber can cause some stomach upset and gurgling sounds while it passes through the colon.

Maintain or achieve a healthy body weight.

Choose 5 or more servings of fruits and vegetables each day.

Limit your intake of saturated and Trans fat and cholesterol.

TIA

short-term prognosis

the risk of stroke after TIA is the highest in the weeks and the months immediately following the event and then decreases with time.

Long-term prognosis:

have a higher incidence of stroke if there is carotid stenosis. Once treated all the risk factors, the stroke risk is less.

Stroke

short-term prognosis

the recent improvements in the management of stroke risk factors, secondary prevention and treatments made the stroke patients lead to better short-term survival and better recovery. Some non-strategic strokes the patients fully recover and forget that even that they had a stroke in the past. Many people with silent strokes or small lacunar strokes of less than 1cm size and non-strategic in location never even know that they had a stroke until incidental imaging study of the brain done and makes them evident on the scans. But many silent strokes together can cause cognitive and physical slowing over time as a combined effect. It is called silent ischemic white matter disease and cognitive impairment.

Long-term prognosis

depends on the strategic location of the stroke and the severity of the consequences.

Depends on the initial residual capabilities of the persons to participate in medical, therapeutic approaches and physical/occupational therapies to improve the functional outcome of stroke in the long run.

Treating underlying medical, surgical causes and maintaining good secondary prevention approaches are most beneficial.

Alzheimer's Dementia, Memory problems

Is gradual impairment of memory and cognition that interferes with a person's work and social relationships.

Several types and Causes are recognized, and some are reversible including depression causing dementia.

Alzheimer's dementia is the most common. The most common warning signs are,

Memory loss, difficulty performing routine tasks, problems with language, disorientation to time and place, abstract thinking problems, misplacing things, poor or decreased judgment, changes in mood, behavior, personality, loss of Initiative qualities.

The 3 stages of Alzheimer's are the cognitive decline, Functional decline and behavioral decline substantially in the last 3 years of the person's life.

Goals of treatment are to stabilize the cognitive impairment and improve the behavioral symptoms.

Medications available mostly are cholinesterase and others.

Future of Alzheimer's therapies

Hoping that during the next 10 years, significant advances will result in both early detection as well as in therapy. Comprehensive care seems essential.

Future for Alzheimer's treatments:

The complexity of Alzheimer's clearly present a challenge to patients, clinicians and researchers.

Continued research geared to uncovering the biology of these disorders through neuroimaging and genetics offers hope for better understanding and treatment.

Diet Mind for Alzheimer's and other dementia/ Memory loss

Adequate sleep is extremely essential for dementia/memory loss persons.

Make sure not having any sleep apnea, thyroid disorders, vitamin deficiencies that can be corrected quickly so their memory can be improved.

If all medical problems managed well if not able to sleep well still explore the possibility of depression on top of dementia and also treat that well.

If still sleep is an issue trying different safe hypnotics will benefit. Avoid the Over the counter Sleep aids that can adversely affect the memory and dementia issues.

Once sleep is addressed, adequate daily sunshine and intellectual stimulation is most important for memory cell activation. Expose to the Sun in the morning at least before the noon for 1 hour.

Daily make a habit of looking at the familiar and favorite things, photos, places, people with in your home and surroundings. President Ronald Reagan did not forget the White House Image even at the later stages of his dementia because it imprinted so strong impression in his brain.

Try to read as much as possible, and especially try to learn a foreign language of your interest, this is a powerful stimulant for the memory cells.

Avoid head injuries, falls that hit head, even trivial head concussions can lead to further memory decline.

Avoid heated arguments, emotional conversations, they will derail the thought process and takes time for the memory to get assembled to baseline.

Persons or family try to postpone the distressing news, emotional news for 6 -7 days to either convey or to act on that news. This will help not only to take appropriate decision but also helps not to derail the existing memory pathways. The roadblocks created each time will further damage the memory cells and memory process to a further extent.

Travelling is good for early dementia/memory loss patients. It stimulates the thought process just like learning a new language, and the persons see different people, different cultures, and surroundings. brain still absorbs the things like a sponge and stimulates the whole memory process.

Long trips that involve closed spaces may be troublesome for dementia persons.

Do not do anything to the extent of physical exhaustion. The body that is physically exhausted takes a toll on the mental energy and makes the memory derailment. Activity is good as permitted. gradual endurance for physical activity is always good.

Remember the principle of Good healthy body is Good brain and healthy brain in the healthy body is the definition of health.

Take all your medications regularly. Some with plenty of fluids, some with food, fallow the druggist instructions.

Keep self-reminders than someone else reminding your appointments, activities. Be active, motivate your self or family member should motivate you, to participate in daily activities to polish and keep up your skills.

Frustration is common for everyone, but keep it off because dementia makes the frustration worse and frustration makes the derailment of memory more and for a longer period to recuperate.

Have small pets like birds, fish, and turtles and watch their moments, listen to their sounds.

Play computer games, or handheld device games on a daily basis.

Recall that day events as the day goes on.

Diet Plate for Alzheimer's dementia/ Memory loss

Avoid alcohol altogether. Or limit to 1 drink every alternate day equal to 1 oz of wine

Have plenty of milk and eat some chocolate daily if can tolerate. Recent research is mentioning that both milk and chocolate can sharpen the memory.

Limit caffeine or tea, but ok to use moderately, some studies showed it may aid memory.

Take multivitamin with essential minerals once a day. Especially treat if any vitamin deficiencies existing. Including B12, Vitamin D contributes to memory decline. Mega vitamins are not capable and in some cases can cause undesirable hypervitaminosis related side effects.

Females if need hormone replacement discuss with your doctor.

Males with testosterone deficiency can include memory issues and can be treated appropriately.

Eat fresh foods, dairy as tolerated. Preserved foods if possible should be avoided or eliminated from regular dietary habits.

Keep yourself well hydrated as much as can tolerate based on your health issues.

Don't forget to eat regularly. Family or caregivers may need to help feed the person well at regular times.

Regular bedtimes, avoiding both advanced or delayed sleep times is particularly useful. The traditional bed sleep times for People with dementia and memory issues are 10 PM to 6.30 AM. (Giving regular 7-8 hours of sleep).

Good foods containing nuts, fruits citrus, almonds, beans, leafy vegetables, omega 3 include foods or capsules are preferred. Keep total calories around 2000 /day.

In summary do enjoy a wide variety of nutritious foods by eating at least three meals every day. Drink plenty of water, prefer to eat plenty of vegetables (including legumes) and fruit. Have plenty of cereals, bread and pastas Eat a diet low in saturated fats. Choose foods low in salt and use salt sparingly. Include foods high in calcium Use added sugars only in moderation.

Dementia Meditation

Morning is the best time for meditation.

After daily activities of living. Look at around in the house at all your familiar pictures, family member's albums once a day.

Interact with the family members if any in the house.

Sit down for meditation session.

Do as Long as can but half an hour to one hour is enough.

Go for a walk or work.

If no other activities planned for the day, solve some puzzles, reading, try to learn a foreign language, play computer games.

Your meditation should increase your concentration and retaining your memory gradually.

Alzheimer's dementia/ memory issues

Short-term prognosis

Secondary causes of memory if treated will improve so well.

Many with the mild cognitive issues may not progress into severe memory loss.

Up to 75% of persons with Alzheimer's disease ultimately are placed in nursing homes where they live for an average of three years at the end stage.

The survival of dementia patients outside the nursing home is better probably due to differences in disease severity.

Patients with the associated psychiatric symptoms of hallucinations, delusions independent of cognitive status may have a rapid functional decline.

Long-term prognosis

the mean length of time from dementia onset to death can range from 5 to 18 years. Due to other co- morbid conditions, the survival can be shortened, but overall length of disease is a relatively poor predictor of clinical course.

Parkinson's Disease: Commonly called PD
&
Tremor

Parkinson's Disease: Commonly called PD

: Is the second most common neurodegenerative disorder (effects the Basal ganglia)in the U.S. after Alzheimer's disease. Common disorder of the elderly but can affect younger individuals also.

Main features are Resting Tremor, Rigidity, and Slowing of the movements and facial expressions. In advanced cases memory also gets impaired in some. All Tremors and shakes are not PD your doctors can help to diagnose benign versus Parkinson's tremor.

Famous People with Parkinson's disease:

Adolph Hitler- Still a subject of debate, but likely suffered from Parkinson's disease.

Mohamed Ali-- a boxer suffered from Parkinson's disease.

Pope John Paul - suffered from Parkinson's disease.

Future of PD

Individuals with Parkinson's disease and society as a whole have a hope for the future. A cure for Parkinson's disease is most likely in the foreseeable future. New research continues to have a positive impact upon society.

Parkinson's, Tremor, Rigidity

Diet Mind:

Tell to yourself that many other better ways of treatments and new medicines, including stem cell, genetic therapies are on the way and may not suffer like this in future. Don't lose hope and trust in modern health sciences

Unfortunately if, depression supervenes, there are many medicines, much needed help and therapies are available.

Maintain a daily routine, Sit up in the bed while trying to get out of bed every day in the morning for 5 minutes with legs hanging down from the side of the bed.

Start your day with your medicines after brushing.

Eat regularly, adequately, better if can.

Treat constipation as needed.

Start your day generously but slowly,

Try to walk as straight as can and watch your arm swing consciously.

Use your vision queues often, I mean does not just walk looking at the front or straight, but create work to your extra ocular muscles(eye muscles) by looking around while walking.

Also, many times try to stop and walk swiftly, stop and turn around as part of your daily routine even though not required to stop or even no body calling from behind. These are easy exercises and will tune your body to over come the Parkinson's effects of making less agile.

If you have tremor and medicines helping or not, practice meditation briefly for 10 minutes Up to 3 times per day. Each time keep the hands straight in front of you, in the air with palms up for 5 minutes and palms down for 5 minutes. This helps to maintain the posture and regulate the tremor and helps the tremor not to get worse with activity.

Walk as much as can. If back is stiff and achy despite adequate doses of medicines that you are on, you may need some pain medication or muscle relaxer along with exercises.

Maintain regular sleep time but do not go to bed too early, do not stay in bed if not sleepy, makes it stiffer Mobility is the best so when you think can go into sleep in next 15- 30 minutes, then only approach the bedroom.

Regular activity, as much as can do are the best way.

Parkinson's patients will have high metabolic rate and calorie burning and may get low in total albumin proteins and vitamins easily leading to deficiencies, malnutrition, weight loss. Parkinson's patients frequently complain about loss of appetite, nausea, weight loss, constipation, drooling slowing of swallow function.

Take medicines regularly.

Brain Diet

Have a well balanced **diet** with the utmost emphasis on high intake of fruits, vegetables, legumes, whole grains, poultry, and fish.

The medication levodopa-dopa usually works best when taken on an empty stomach about ½ hour before meals or at least one hour after meals. It should be taken with plenty of water. This allows the drug to absorb more quickly.

Drink clear or ice-cold drinks.

Avoid orange and grapefruit juices, because these are too acidic and may worsen nausea.

Drink beverages slowly but plenty.

Drink liquids between meals instead of during meals.

Eat light, bland foods (such as saltine crackers or plain bread).

Avoid fried, greasy, or sugary foods.

Eat slowly.

Eat smaller, more frequent meals throughout the day.

Eat foods that are cold or at room temperature to avoid getting nauseated from the smell of hot or warm foods.

Rest after eating, keeping your head elevated. Activity may worsen nausea and may lead to vomiting.

Avoid brushing your teeth after eating to prevent gagging and vomiting.

Try to eat when feel less nauseated.

Limit caffeine beverages contained in coffee, tea, cola, and chocolate as it may interfere with some of your medications and may actually produce more dehydrated, may worsen your tremor.

Take a sip of liquid after each bite to moisten your mouth and help swallow.

Eat sour candy, fruit or chew ice to help increase saliva and moisten your mouth.

Avoid non-nutritious beverages.

Eat small, frequent meals and snacks.

Walk or participate in another light activity to stimulate your appetite.

Plan meals to include your favorite foods.

Try eating the high-calorie foods in your meal first.

Use your imagination to increase the variety of food.

Choose high-protein and high-calorie snacks. High calorie snacks include ice cream, cookies, pudding, cheese, granola bars, custard, sandwiches, nachos with cheese, eggs, crackers with peanut butter, bagels with peanut butter or cream cheese, cereal fruit or vegetables with dips, yogurt with granola, popcorn with margarine and parmesan cheese, or bread sticks with cheese sauce.

Brain diet

Malnutrition and weight maintenance are often an issue for people with Parkinson's disease. Here are some tips to help you maintain a healthy weight.

Weigh yourself once or twice a week.

If you have any ongoing weight gain or loss like 2 pounds in one day or 5 pounds in one week contact your doctor.

To gain weight.

Take nutritional supplements in the form of snacks, drinks as Ensure or Boost, may be prescribed to eat between meals to help increase your calories and get the right amount of nutrients every day.

Use whole milk, whole milk cheese, and yogurt. Try to get most of your protein from legumes, beans, soy and fish. focus mostly on poultry with an occasional serving of red meat. have a high protein diet,

Avoid artificial sweeteners and preservatives include aspartame and monosodium glutamate.

Avoid alcohol, sugar and caffeine, all can disrupt neurological function. Also try to avoid any type of processed food that contains high levels of chemicals and toxins.

PD/Tremor Meditation

Do morning balance and coordination exercises first.

After activities of daily living, do meditation for half an hour to 1 hour.

Use any comfortable position.

Lot of Parkinson's patients get spine stiffness with back spasms in anyone position after a short time.

Meditation along with later exercise programs will help to coordinate the moments better, decreases body spasms, stiffness and helps their memory and sleep.

Parkinson's disease

short-term prognosis

Depends on how the person responds to L-dopa. In general that fail to respond to this drug will not significantly respond to another anti-Parkinson's medications in any significant way.

Now a days deep brain stimulation is available for only those who respond well to L-dopa too.

Long-term prognosis

Is not good but is highly variable. Future will change this with new treatment keep coming.

The death rate is probably lower with L-dopa than without it.

This is a progressive disease with changes and the decline in the substantia nigra cell population in the brain. Also, the response to the anti Parkinson's medicines slowly becomes less and less.

Progression is equal for men and women but is slower in-patients with early disease onset and in those with the prominent tremor.

Dementia occurs in a more than 30% to 50% of PD patients.

The dementia progression is as variable as is the motor dysfunction but generally mental decline parallels the physical decline.

Essential tremor

short-term prognosis

Usually if, mild and made worse by stress, treatment may not be indicated.

Very slowly progressive in most patients. Overall favorable prognosis.

Long-term prognosis

In some patients, all forms of treatment eventually will fail, and Deep brain stimulation can be highly useful with success rates of as high as 85% to control the tremor consistently.

Most patients with the essential tremor any way will not experience such a poor quality of life.

Multiple Sclerosis

well known as MS, this is a chronic demyelinating disease of the brain and cervical spine of unknown etiology. The manifestations are extremely variable in type and severity.

Diagnosis: Based on Clinical features, spinal tap(lumbar puncture) MRI brain scan, eye exam and rarely others called VEP and SSPE's are used to diagnose and monitor the condition. Onset usually between 20-40. The Goal of treatment is to shorten and decrease the frequency of attacks and keep the person functional.

Future treatments for MS

Over the last 2 decades the treatments for Multiple Sclerosis has evolved rapidly. There are even more ideas. One such idea is to prevent the degeneration of axons and/or promote Remyelination. Oral therapy is available now, and many other oral agents coming soon into the market that would be a change from self-injection therapy.

Multiple Sclerosis/ Spasticity

Remember It is rare for MS to take away your speech, swallow, special senses.

In few, it may cause some cognitive difficulties.

Overall it is a terrible disease but will not cripple your higher mental capabilities.

The troubles that MS persons get into are sudden episodic Blindness, weakness by involving the brain and spinal card.

Fatigue, muscle spasms, stiffness, gait disability, bladder and bowel dysfunction can happen.

Rare, but aggressive cases can cause cognitive issues, cripples the person to bed bound state.

If you are reading this you should be happy that there is a hope and a lot of new medications and research is on going.

Diet Mind

Go to sleep regularly and get up at regular time. This very important as per not making your body and muscles stiffer.

Use a comfortable but firm bed (Not too soft or too Hard).

If possible use headboard to rest your head along with a firm pillow or comfortable pillow.

Sleep only as needed. Because of fatigue, feel like staying in the bed but come out of the bed with effort and stay out of the bed after bedtime.

Try to stay away from coffee, tea, any energy drinks and over the counter stimulants.

Stay away from diet beverages. Tobacco and any other brain stimulant or altering agents including marijuana.

Prefer orange or apple juice.

Eat high fiber diet, plenty of fluids and regular water.

Stretch your body frequently from side to side and each extremity at a time. Yoga, Tai chi can help you how to relax and stretch and mould your body to prevent spasms.

walk as much as can daily until fatigue supervenes.

There are some good medicines that can help your fatigue.

Try to do house hold or other daily activity as much as you can. More activity is good.

Take warm bath twice a day. MS persons have intolerance to heat/temperature, but warm bath can be soothing.

Avoid constipation by taking plenty of fluids, fiber containing foods.

Try to avoid routine use of Sleep aids especially over the counter which cause next day more fatigue.

Brain Diet

Try to Become mostly vegetarian with diet by eating less animal food (meat, chicken, eggs, dairy, etc.) and more plant-based foods (such as fruits, vegetables, beans, legumes, nuts, seeds, whole grains, whole soy) and the fish.

Although fish is an animal food, fish is extremely low in saturated fat and also has important anti-inflammatory omega-3 fats. plant based foods are good not only just fruits and vegetables. You'll find phytonutrients in nuts, seeds, whole grains, beans, legumes, whole soy, etc. Each day eat fruit with breakfast and vegetables with both lunch and dinner.

Less oil and more spices are ok (such as turmeric, cinnamon, cumin and cardamom). And it is not just spices, but herbs are also a very healthy way to add flavor to your food.

Avoid food made with refined flour of any sort (if it is "enriched" it is processed). Avoid any food with high fructose corn syrup and eat sugar only in moderation. However, good "whole carbohydrates" are extremely healthy and not only are packed with fiber and a broad spectrum of vitamins and minerals, but they also contain lots of phytonutrients. "Good" whole carbs to eat daily include fruits, vegetables, beans, legumes, corn, whole grains, sprouted whole grain breads and sprouted whole grain pastas.

Avoid Trans Fats. There is no safe level of intake for Trans fats. Trans fats increase inflammation, decrease sensitivity to insulin, increase your LDL cholesterol, decrease your good HDL cholesterol, impair artery dilation, and increase your triglyceride levels. Whether you are on a diet for multiple sclerosis or not, you should eat zero grams of Trans fats per day.

MS meditation

Do meditation in the morning 1/2 to 1 hour after regular stretching exercises.

If possible do meditation in the evening also, so total of two sessions per day is good.

Any comfortable position is okay to do meditation.

Multiple sclerosis

short-term prognosis

is palatable for most MS patients.

At the onset, only a small minority show acute fulminate course.

Long-term prognosis

The majority eventually develops a disability at least a 50% of relapsing patients enter a secondary progressive stage.

30% of progressive patients stabilize for several years and a small portion even may show improvement.

Migraines & Headaches

are several types and most are benign but severe nagging in pain. Takes the quality of life from the sufferers. It costs so many productive working days and makes the person irritable, distracted, depressed too. All new onset, thunderclap, severe headaches need immediate attention. Fortunately so many new medications available to control the headaches that are both acute and chronic in nature.

Once serious conditions that cause headaches are ruled out further treatment depends on the frequency, severity and the nature of headaches whether they are tension type, migraines, migraine variants, rarely cluster type headaches or other like related to neck pain and arthritis, scalp sensitivity issues.

As per treatment includes controlling the triggers if any identified, avoiding the agents that precipitate the headaches(prevention is better than cure). Then there are further preventive or prophylactic agents or abortive agents for the headaches.

Famous people with migraines

Historical Figures suffered with headaches are

Thomas Jefferson: (April 13, 1743 – July 4, 1826) was an American Founding Father, the principal author of the Declaration of Independence (1776) and the third President of the United states (1801–1809).

Julius Caesar :(July 100 BC – 15 March 44 BC) was a Roman general, statesman, Consul and notable author of Latin prose.

Napoleon Bonaparte: (15 August 1769 – 5 May 1821) was a French military and political leader who rose to prominence during the latter stages of the French Revolution and its associated wars in Europe. As Napoleon I, he was Emperor of the French from 1804 to 1815.

Ulysses S. Grant: (April 27, 1822 – July 23, 1885) was the 18th President of the United States (1869–1877) following his highly successful role as a war general in the second half of the Civil War.

Robert Edward Lee: (January 19, 1807 – October 12, 1870) was a career military officer who is best known for having commanded the Confederate Army of Northern Virginia in the American Civil War.

Vincent van Gogh: (30 March 1853 – 29 July 1890) was a Dutch post-Impressionist painter.

Sigmund Freud: (6 May 1856 – 23 September 1939) was an Austrian neurologist who became known as the founding father of psychoanalysis.

Elvis Presley: (January 8, 1935 – August 16, 1977) was an American singer and actor. A cultural icon, he is commonly known by the single name Elvis. One of the most popular musicians of the 20th century, he is often referred to as the "King of Rock and Roll" or "the King".

Many famous Athletes also suffer from headaches.

Migraine headaches are quite common among neurologists who ironically treat that condition.

Famous people are no different from any of the rest of us when it comes to migraines, but it can be reassuring to see what people have been able to accomplish despite having episodic debilitating condition. Perhaps you can get some encouragement as you consider how many people were affected by migraine headaches. There are many medications available to treat and prevent migraines. But each patient may need to try up to 5 different preventive agents before they find the right agent for them that prevents their migraines. By the way, lot of research says the medications are only 50% better than the placebo effect. So by avoiding triggers, maintaining, good sleep habits and time management will help to treat and avoid headaches.

Future of Migraines

I guess new medications may come for better, quicker relief of headaches, with staying away from narcotics as a goal, but no specific therapies to solve the headache altogether and forever may not be in the pipeline. No gene therapies either. Still all the medications that are used for migraine prophylaxis are only 50% better than placebo agents. This means lot of headaches are controlled by controlling the triggers and maintaining harmony of body & mind and controlling the social stresses as much as one can.

Migraine Diet

Diet Mind for Migraine

First know the truth and myth about your migraine. Like lots of sinus headaches are migraines infect rather than sinus headaches themselves.

Make sure that no serious reason exists for your headaches by brain scans.

Make sure that do not have any other medical reasons like sinus disease or connective tissue disease to cause those headaches.

Then find the triggers for your headaches and eliminate if find one like

Strong odors, smells perfume, sounds, glaring lights, and environmental allergens.

Eliminate the foods that trigger your migraines like MSG, chocolate, some spices, diet drinks, alcohol, substitute sugars, some meat products and many.

You have to screen your self with all the foods that you are exposed, to find that single food that bothers you with headaches. Some persons are allergic and intolerant to very unusual and unexpected common food items that no body considers them as a trigger.

Sleep disturbance, lack of restful sleep are one main reason for migraines.

Anticipated anxiety, depression is another key reason for migraines.

Compulsive nature, obsessive nature, types "A" personalities get most migraines.

Behavioral modification, meditation will help migraines.

Migraine patients most are either too busy, aggressive professionally or on a daily basis worry a lot and ruminate on same worrisome thoughts with little physical activity.

Regular scheduled activity, punctuality with their daily living activities and day to day life will help migraines.

Adequate sleep (not over sleeping) will help migraines.

Using headboard with comfortable pillow will help migraines.

Acupuncture likely will help migraines.

Creating pressure by your own finger tips, small plastic, wood devices on the occipital and scalp nerves to create pressure on a daily basis for 15-30 minutes will help migraines too. This is called trigger point stimulation.

Avoid the triggers like bright lights, computer screens, moving light, chocolate and other foods.

Wines especially red wine cause lots of migraines, Overall avoid all alcoholic and stimulant drinks but if must drink on occasions chose vodka which is least likely in small quantities to cause

Migraine. Some tolerate specific wines carefully chosen over many years of self-experience by trial and error.

Control the migraine triggers including (in women) the hormonal changes prior to menstruation.

Changes in weather, lack of sleep, stress, and skipping meals can all bring on the headaches.

Aerobic exercise daily will help.

Meditation, Yoga, Tai chi, daily will help.

Brain Diet for Migraine

Avoid Tyramine, Aged cheese, MSG, chocolate and other food triggers like mentioned above.

Avoid foods that cause constipation. Straining at the toilet is another strong trigger for migraine.

Don't skip meals.

Do not get to the stage that are truly hungry, that is a migraine trigger.

Sexual headaches with excitement and exertion headaches needs good rehydration, avoid anticipatory anxiety regarding oncoming headache, start slow any exertion, maintain the tempo and end gradually without stopping suddenly.

Low calorie, low refined sugars, low fatty, greasy foods will help migraines.

For foods that involve vigorous chewing, make sure to use both sides of jaws. Lot of people prefers one side than other and routinely chew food on one side of the jaw only either right or left. This provokes triggering the Trigeminal ganglion and migraine pathways with TMJ like symptoms with migraines.

Avoid Aspartame (Equal, NutraSweet), other artificial sweeteners, foods with meat tenderizers or yeast and yeast extracts.

Caffeine in even in small amounts can trigger a migraine in some people. Lot of medicines that we use to treat acute headache does contain caffeine and help for headache relief too.

Chocolate, cocoa, and foods containing nuts, alcoholic beverages especially red wine, beer, and Aged, canned, cured, or processed meats such as chicken livers and other organ meats, and sardines can cause headaches.

Also, foods prepared with nitrates or tyramine can cause problems.

Cultured dairy products such as sour cream or buttermilk, dried fruits including figs, raisins, and dates, Breads and crackers containing cheese including pizza, Cheese Smoked or dried fish and Canned soups can trigger your migraines too.

So overall screen by trial and error and find all the triggers for your headaches and avoid them once see them as a trigger.

Prefer To eat

Plenty of purple grape juice is beneficial.

Fresh and raw vegetables are no harm.

Weekly twice meat in limited quantities is ok.

Dried fruits, nuts.

Snacks ok without aged cheese and not much refined sugars.

Prefer citrus, apple and other fresh juices.

Ripe bananas 1-2 /day. contains Serotonin, may help some with migraines with its calming and soothing effect. If you do not like or allergic to bananas ok to void.

The best foods for magnesium include spinach, potatoes, sunflower seeds, and whole grains and other. We use magnesium to treat migraines.

Cereal with milk if not lactose intolerant, plenty of water, low fat and unsaturated fatty foods to prefer.

Migraine and Meditation

work on stress relief, ruminating thoughts, intrusive thoughts, causing your migraine headaches.

Do meditation two times once in AM and at bedtime.

When woke up in the morning stay in bed for 10 minutes in a relaxed state.

Imagine the day without the stress and headache.

After daily activities of living if no time just go to work.

In the mid-day try to relax 15 to 30 minutes either with a brief nap or meditation.

Just sit and relax quite and calm forgetting worries and pain.

In the evening maintain a dedicated half-hour session for meditation and the standard position if possible.

Do it regularly and do not give up. You'll see many benefits not only getting rid of headaches.

Migraine

short-term prognosis

varies and depends on each patient's proper use of medications, avoiding triggers, controlling any psychological factors contributing to headaches.

The response to prophylactic agents does not exceed 50% than placebo.

Long-term prognosis

So far cure for migraine does not exist. Majority will enjoy the self-limited nature and the tendency for attenuation of headaches over time.

Individualizing therapy for those with the medical, psychiatric, neurological co-morbidity seems to be important.

Conclusion

We all need to stay healthy, functional, and happy forever. We do not ask for illness. When it comes like an evil, we don't have a choice, other than facing it. Then, we have to use all available resources. Respecting the body, we need to treat it well with ideal dietary choices, take all medications regularly, exercise adequately and keep ourselves occupied in all possible ways. Practicing daily without giving up is most beneficial.

If not your choice until now, it could be yours now. Your goals do not have any deadline to ensure the best possible results. You are that Anybody, Somebody and Everybody. But 'Nobody' any more. Take a plunge and change yourself to reach your potential.

INDEX